SpringerBriefs in Statistics

More information about this series at http://www.springer.com/series/8921

Ton J. Cleophas · Aeilko H. Zwinderman

Machine Learning in Medicine—Cookbook Three

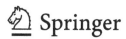 Springer

Ton J. Cleophas
Department of Medicine
Albert Schweitzer Hospital
Sliedrecht
The Netherlands

Aeilko H. Zwinderman
Department of Biostatistics and
  Epidemiology
Academic Medical Center
Leiden
The Netherlands

Additional material to this book can be downloaded from http://extras.springer.com/

ISSN 2191-544X   ISSN 2191-5458 (electronic)
ISBN 978-3-319-12162-8   ISBN 978-3-319-12163-5 (eBook)
DOI 10.1007/978-3-319-12163-5

Library of Congress Control Number: 2013957369

Springer Cham Heidelberg New York Dordrecht London

Printed on acid-free paper

Springer is part of Springer Science+Business Media (www.springer.com)

Preface

The amount of medical data is estimated to double every 20 months, and clinicians are at a loss to analyze them. Fortunately, user friendly statistical software has been helpful for the past 30 years. However, traditional statistical methods have difficulty to identify outliers in large datasets, and to find patterns in big data and data with multiple exposure/outcome variables. In addition, analysis-rules for surveys and questionnaires, which are currently common methods of medical data collection, are, essentially, missing. Fortunately, a new discipline, machine learning, is able to cover all of these limitations. It involves computationally intensive methods like factor analysis, cluster analysis, and discriminant analysis. It is currently mainly the domain of computer scientists, and is already commonly used in social sciences, marketing research, operational research, and applied sciences. It is little used in medical research, probably due to the traditional belief of clinicians in clinical trials where multiple variables even out by the randomization process, and are not taken into account. In contrast, modern medical computer files often involve hundreds of variables like genes and other laboratory values, and computationally intensive methods are required.

In the past 2 years we have completed a series of three textbooks entitled *Machine Learning in Medicine Part One, Two, and Three* (ed. by Springer Heidelberg Germany, 2012–2013). Also, we produced two-100 page cookbooks, entitled *Machine Learning in Medicine—Cookbook One and Two*. These cookbooks were

(1) without background information and theoretical discussions,
(2) highlighting technical details,
(3) with data examples available at extras.springer.com for readers to perform their own analyses,
(4) with references to the above textbooks for those wishing background information.

The current volume, entitled *Machine Learning in Medicine—Cookbook Three* was written in a way much similar to that of the first two, and it reviews concised versions of machine learning methods so far, like spectral plots, Bayesian networks, support vector machines (Chaps. 9, 12, 13). Also, a first description is given of several new methods already employed by technical and market scientists, and of their suitabilities for clinical research, like ordinal scalings for inconsistent intervals, loglinear models for varying incident risks, iteration methods for cross-validations (Chaps. 4–6, 16).

Additional new subjects are the following. Chapter 1 describes a novel method for data mining using visualization processes instead of calculus methods. Chapter 2 describes the use of trained clusters, a scientifically more appropriate alternative for traditional cluster analysis. Chapter 11 describes evolutionary operations (evops), and the evop calculators, already widely used in chemical and technical process improvements.

Similar to the first cookbook, the current work will assess in a nonmathematical way the stepwise analyses of 20 machine learning methods, that are, likewise, based on three major machine learning methodologies:

Cluster Methodologies (Chaps. 1, 2),
Linear Methodologies (Chaps. 3–8),
Rules Methodologies (Chaps. 9–20).

In extras.springer.com the data files of the examples (14 SPSS files) are given (both real and hypothesized data). Furthermore, 4 csv type excel files are available for data analysis in the Konstanz Information Miner, a widely approved free machine learning software package on the Internet since 2006.

The current 100-page book entitled *Machine Learning in Medicine—Cookbook Three*, and its complementary "Cookbooks One and Two" are written as training companions for 60 important machine learning methods relevant to medicine. We should emphasize that all of the methods described have been successfully applied in the authors' own research.

Lyon, August 2014   Ton J. Cleophas
                                                                      Aeilko H. Zwinderman

Contents of Previous Volumes

Machine Learning in Medicine—Cookbook One

Machine Learning in Medicine—Cookbook Two

Contents

Part II   Linear Models

Part I
Cluster Models

Chapter 1
Data Mining for Visualization of Health Processes (150 Patients with Pneumonia)

1.1 General Purpose

Computer files of clinical data are often complex and multi-dimensional, and they are, frequently, hard to statistically test. Instead, visualization processes can be successfully used as an alternative approach to traditional statistical data analysis.

For example, Konstanz Information Miner (KNIME) software has been developed by computer scientists from Silicon Valley in collaboration with technicians from Konstanz University at the Bodensee in Switzerland, and it pays particular attention to visual data analysis. It is used since 2006 as a freely available package through the Internet. So far, it is mainly used by chemists and pharmacists, but not by clinical investigators. This chapter is to assess, whether visual processing of clinical data may, sometimes, perform better than traditional statistical analysis.

1.2 Primary Scientific Question

Can visualization processes of clinical data provide insights that remained hidden with traditional statistical tests?

1.3 Example

Four inflammatory markers [C-reactive protein (CRP), erythrocyte sedimentation rate (ESR), leucocyte count (leucos), and fibrinogen)] were measured. In 150 patients with pneumonia. Based on X-ray chest clinical severity was classified as

© The Author(s) 2014
T.J. Cleophas and A.H. Zwinderman, *Machine Learning in Medicine—Cookbook Three*, SpringerBriefs in Statistics,
DOI 10.1007/978-3-319-12163-5_1

A (mild infection), B (medium severity), C (severe infection). One scientific question was to assess whether the markers could adequately predict the severity of infection.

CRP	Leucos'	Fibrinogen	ESR	X-ray severity
120.00	5.00	11.00	60.00	A
100.00	5.00	11.00	56.00	A
94.00	4.00	11.00	60.00	A
92.00	5.00	11.00	58.00	A
100.00	5.00	11.00	52.00	A
108.00	6.00	17.00	48.00	A
92.00	5.00	14.00	48.00	A
100.00	5.00	11.00	54.00	A
88.00	5.00	11.00	54.00	A
98.00	5.00	8.00	60.00	A
108.00	5.00	11.00	68.00	A
96.00	5.00	11.00	62.00	A
96.00	5.00	8.00	46.00	A
86.00	4.00	8.00	60.00	A
116.00	4.00	11.00	50.00	A
114.00	5.00	17.00	52.00	A

CRP C-reactive protein (mg/l)
Leucos leucocyte count (*10^9/l)
Fibrinogen fibrinogen level (mg/l)
ESR erythrocyte sedimentation rate (mm)
X-ray severity X-chest severity pneumonia score (A − C = mild to severe)

The first 15 patients are above. The entire data file is entitled "decision tree", and is available in http://extras.springer.com. Data analysis of these data in SPSS is rather limited. Start by opening the data file in SPSS statistical software.

Command:
click Graphs…Legacy Dialogs…Bar Charts…click Simple…click Define… Category Axis: enter "severity score"…Variable: enter CRP…mark Other statistics…click OK.

After performing the same procedure for the other variables four graphs are produced as shown underneath. The mean levels of all of the inflammatory markers consistently tended to rise with increasing severities of infection. Univariate multinomial logistic regression with severity as outcome gives a significant effect of all of the markers. However, this effect is largely lost in the multiple multinomial logistic regression, probably due to interactions.

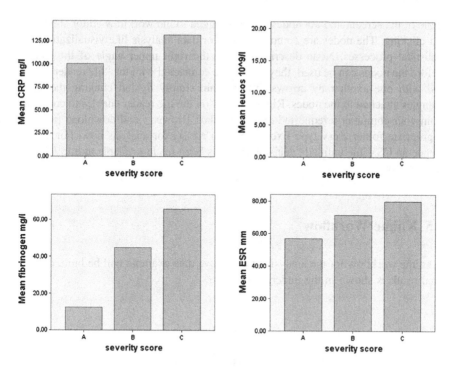

We are interested to explore these results for additional effects, for example, hidden data effects, like different predictive effects and frequency distributions for different subgroups. For that purpose KNIME data miner will be applied. SPSS data files can not be downloaded directly in the KNIME software, but excel files can, and SPSS data can be saved as an excel file (the cvs file type available in your computer must be used).

Command in SPSS:
click File...click Save as...in "Save as" type: enter Comma Delimited (*.csv)... click Save.

1.4 Knime Data Miner

In Google enter the term "knime". Click Download and follow instructions. After completing the pretty easy download procedure, open the knime workbench by clicking the knime welcome screen. The center of the screen displays the workflow editor like the canvas in SPSS Modeler. It is empty, and can be used to build a stream of nodes, called workflow in knime. The node repository is in the left lower angle of the screen, and the nodes can be dragged to the workflow editor simply by left-clicking. The nodes are computer tools for data analysis like visualization and statistical processes. Node description is in the right upper angle of the screen. Before the nodes can be used, they have to be connected with the "file reader" node, and with one another by arrows drawn again simply by left clicking the small triangles attached to the nodes. Right clicking on the file reader enables to configure from your computer a requested data file…click Browse…and download from the appropriate folder a csv type Excel file. You are set for analysis now. For convenience an CSV file entitled "decisiontree" has been made available at http://extras.springer.com.

1.5 Knime Workflow

A knime workflow for the analysis of the above data example will be built, and the final result is shown in the underneath figure.

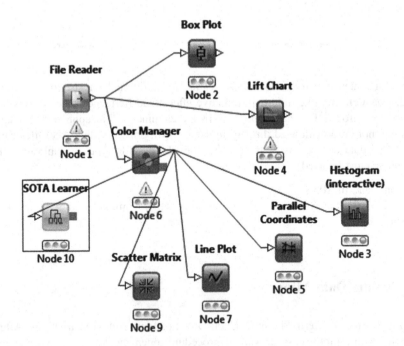

1.6 Box and Whiskers Plots

In the node repository find the node Box Plot. First click the IO option (import/ export option nodes). Then click "Read", then the File Reader node is displayed, and can be dragged by left clicking to the workflow editor. Enter the requested data file as described above. A Node dialog is displayed underneath the node entitled Node 1. Its light is orange at this stage, and should turn green before it can be applied. If you right click the node's center, and then left click File Table a preview of the data is supplied.

Now, in the search box of the node repository find and click Data Views...then "Box plot"...drag to workflow editor...connect with arrow to File reader...right click File reader...right click execute...right click Box Plot node...right click Configurate...right click Execute and open view...

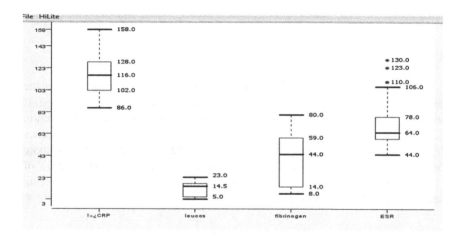

The above box plots with 95 % confidence intervals of the four variable are displayed. The ESR plot shows that also outliers have been displayed. The smallest confidence interval has the leucocyte count, and it may, thus, be the best predictor.

1.7 Lift Chart

In the node repository...click Lift Chart and drag to workflow editor... connect with arrow to File reader...right click execute Lift Chart node...right click Configurate...right click Execute and open view...

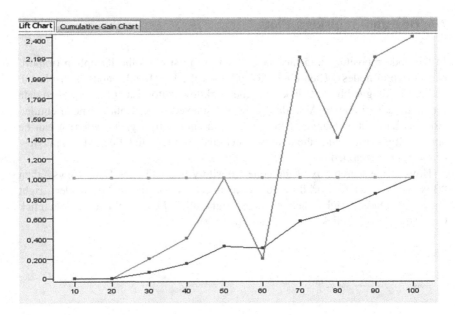

The lift chart shows the predictive performance of the data assuming that the four inflammatory markers are predictors and the severity score is the outcome. If the predictive performance is no better than random, the ratio successful prediction with/without the model = 1.000 (the green line). The x-axis give dociles (1 = 10 = 10 % of the entire sample etc.). It can be observed that at 7 or more dociles the predictive performance start to be pretty good (with ratios of 2.100–2.400. Logistic regression (here multinomial logistic regression) is being used by Knime for making predictions.

1.8 Histogram

In the node repository click type color...click the color manager node and drag to workflow editor...in node repository click color...click the Esc button of your computer...click Data Views...select interactive histogram and transfer to workflow editor...connect color manager node with File Reader...connect color manager with "interactive histogram node"...right click Configurate...right click Execute and open view...

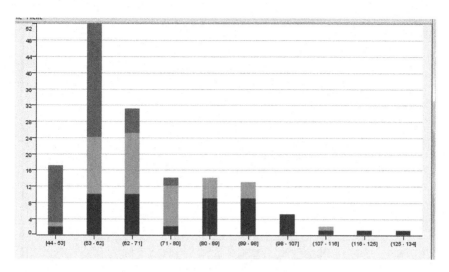

Interactive histograms with bins of ESR values are given. The colors provide the proportions of cases with mild severity (A, red), medium severity (B, green), and severe pneumonias (C, blue). It can be observed that many mild cases (red) are in the ESR 44–71 mm cut-off. Above ESR of 80 mm blue (severe pneumonia) is increasingly present. The software program has selected only the ESR values 44–134. Instead of histograms with ESR, those with other predictor variables can be made.

1.9 Line Plot

In the node repository click Data Views…select the node Line plots and transfer to workflow editor…connect color manager with "Line plots"…right click Configurate…right click Execute and open view…

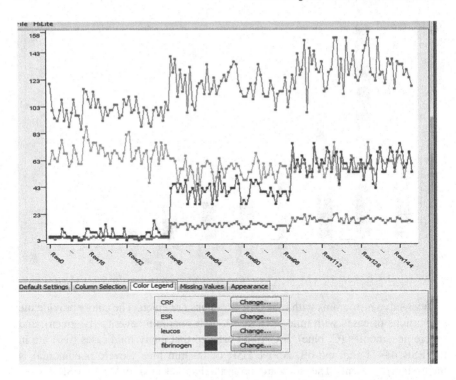

The line plot gives the values of all cases along the x-axis. The upper curve are the CRP values. The middle one the ESR values. The lower part are the leucos and fibrinogen values. The rows 0–50 are the cases with mild pneumonia, the rows 51–100 the medium severity cases, and the rows 101–150 the severe cases. It can be observed that particularly the CRP-, fibrinogen-, and leucos levels increase with increased severity of infection. This is not observed with the ESR levels.

1.10 Matrix of Scatter Plots

In the node repository click Data Views...select "Matrix of scatter plots" and transfer to workflow editor...connect color manager with "Matrix of scatter plots"...right click Configure...right click Execute and open view...

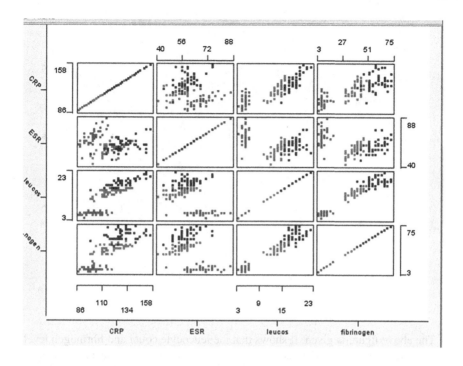

The above figure gives the results. The four predictors variables are plotted against one another. By the colors (blue for severest, red for mildest pneumonias) the fields show that the severest pneumonias are predominantly in the right upper quadrant, the mildest in the left lower quadrant.

1.11 Parallel Coordinates

In the node repository click Data Views...select "Parallel coordinates" and transfer to workflow editor...connect color manager with "Parallel coordinates" ...right click Configurate...right click Execute and open view...click Appearance...click Draw (spline) Curves instead of lines...

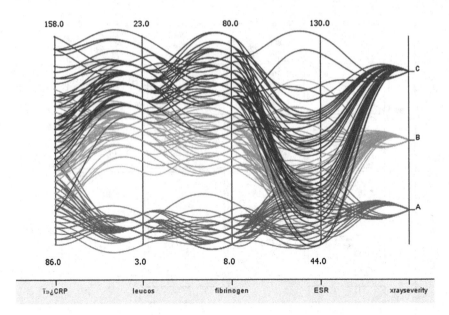

The above figure is given. It shows that the leucocyte count and fibrinogen level are excellent predictors of infection severities. CRP and ESR are also adequate predictors of infections with mild and medium severities, however, poor predictors of levels of severe infections.

1.12 Hierarchical Cluster Analysis with SOTA (Self Organizing Tree Algorithm)

In the node repository click Mining...select the node Self Organizing tree Algorithm (SOTA) Learner and transfer to workflow editor...connect color manager with "SOTA learner"...right click Configurate...right click Execute and open view...

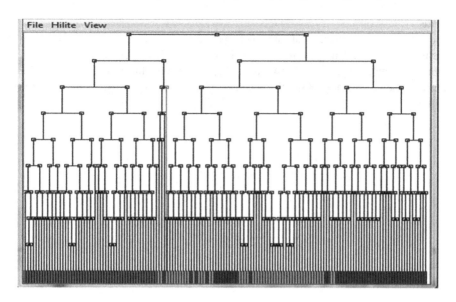

SOTA learning is a modified hierarchical cluster analysis, and it uses in this example the between-case distances of fibrinogen as variable. On the y-axis are standardized distances of the cluster combinations. Clicking the small squares interactively demonstrates the row numbers of the individual cases. It can be observed at the bottom of the figure that the severity classes very well cluster, with the mild cases (red) left, medium severity (green) in the middle, and severe cases (blue) right.

1.13 Conclusion

Clinical computer files are complex, and hard to statistically test. Instead, visualization processes can be successfully used as an alternative approach to traditional statistical data analysis. For example, KNIME (Konstanz Information Miner) software developed by computer scientists at Konstanz University Technical Department at the Bodensee, although mainly used by chemists and pharmacists, is able to visualize multidimensional clinical data, and this approach may, sometimes, perform better than traditional statistical testing. In the current example it was able to demonstrate the clustering of inflammatory markers to identify different classes of pneumonia severity. Also to demonstrate that leucocyte count and fibrinogen were the best markers, and that ESR was a poor marker. In all of the markers the best predictive performance was obtained in the severest cases of disease. All of these observations were unobserved in the traditional statistical analysis in SPSS.

Note

More background, theoretical and mathematical information of splines and hierarchical cluster modeling are in Machine Learning in Medicine Part One, Chap. 11, Non-linear modeling, pp. 127–143, and Chap. 15, Hierarchical cluster analysis for unsupervised data, pp. 183–195, Springer Heidelberg Germany, from the same authors.

Chapter 2
Training Decision Trees for a More Meaningful Accuracy (150 Patients with Pneumonia)

2.1 General Purpose

Traditionally, decision trees are used for finding the best predictors of health risks and improvements (Chap. 16 in Machine Learning in Medicine Cookbook One, pp. 97–104, Decision trees for decision analysis, Springer Heidelberg Germany, 2014, from the same authors). However, this method is not entirely appropriate, because a decision tree is built from a data file, and, subsequently, the same data file is applied once more for computing the health risk probabilities from the built tree. Obviously, the accuracy must be close to 100 %, because the test sample is 100 % identical to the sample used for building the tree, and, therefore, this accuracy does not mean too much. With neural networks this problem of duplicate usage of the same data is solved by randomly splitting the data into two samples, a training sample and a test sample (Chap. 12 in Machine Learning in Medicine Part One, pp. 145–156, Artificial intelligence, multilayer perceptron modeling, Springer Heidelberg Germany, 2013, from the same authors). The current chapter is to assess whether the splitting methodology, otherwise called partitioning, is also feasible for decision trees, and to assess its level of accuracy.

2.2 Primary Scientific Question

Can inflammatory markers adequately predict pneumonia severities with the help of a decision tree. Can partitioning of the data improve the methodology and is sufficient accuracy of the methodology maintained.

© The Author(s) 2014
T.J. Cleophas and A.H. Zwinderman, *Machine Learning in Medicine—Cookbook Three*, SpringerBriefs in Statistics, DOI 10.1007/978-3-319-12163-5_2

2.3 Example

Four inflammatory markers [C-reactive protein (CRP), erythrocyte sedimentation rate (ESR), leucocyte count (leucos), and fibrinogen] were measured in 150 patients. Based on X-ray chest clinical severity was classified as A (mild infection), B (medium severity), C (severe infection). A major scientific question was to assess what markers were the best predictors of the severity of infection.

CRP	Leucos'	Fibrinogen	ESR	X-ray severity
120.00	5.00	11.00	60.00	A
100.00	5.00	11.00	56.00	A
94.00	4.00	11.00	60.00	A
92.00	5.00	11.00	58.00	A
100.00	5.00	11.00	52.00	A
108.00	6.00	17.00	48.00	A
92.00	5.00	14.00	48.00	A
100.00	5.00	11.00	54.00	A
88.00	5.00	11.00	54.00	A
98.00	5.00	8.00	60.00	A
108.00	5.00	11.00	68.00	A
96.00	5.00	11.00	62.00	A
96.00	5.00	8.00	46.00	A
86.00	4.00	8.00	60.00	A
116.00	4.00	11.00	50.00	A
114.00	5.00	17.00	52.00	A

CRP C-reactive protein (mg/l)
Leucos leucocyte count ($*10^9$ /l)
Fibrinogen fibrinogen level (mg/l)
ESR erythrocyte sedimentation rate (mm)
X-ray severity X-chest severity pneumonia score (A − C = mild to severe)

The first 16 patients are in the above table, the entire data file is in "decision tree" and can be obtained from "http://extras.springer.com" on the internet. We will start by opening the data file in SPSS.

Command:
click Classify…Tree…Dependent Variable: enter severity score…Independent Variables: enter CRP, Leucos, fibrinogen, ESR…Growing Method: select CHAID…click Output: mark Tree in table format…Criteria: Parent Node type 50, Child Node type 15…click Continue… …click OK.

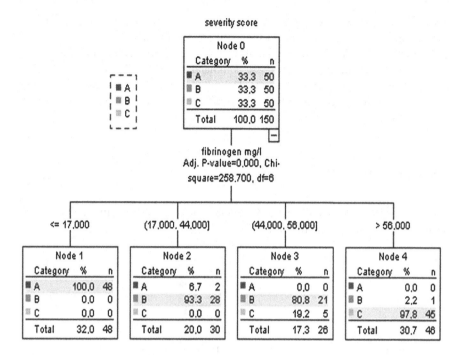

The above decision tree is displayed. A fibrinogen level <17 is 100 % predictor of severity score A (mild disease). Fibrinogen 17–44 gives 93 % chance of severity B, fibrinogen 44–56 gives 81 % chance of severity B, and fibrinogen >56 gives 98 % chance of severity score C. The output also shows that the overall accuracy of the model is 94.7 %, but we have to account that this model is somewhat flawed, because all of the data are used twice, one, for building the tree, and, second, for using the tree for making predictions.

2.4 Downloading the Knime Data Miner

In Google enter the term "knime". Click Download and follow instructions. After completing the pretty easy download procedure, open the knime workbench by clicking the knime welcome screen. The center of the screen displays the workflow editor. Like the canvas in SPSS Modeler, it is empty, and can be used to build a stream of nodes, called workflow in knime. The node repository is in the left lower angle of the screen, and the nodes can be dragged to the workflow editor simply by left-clicking. The nodes are computer tools for data analysis like visualization and statistical processes. Node description is in the right upper angle of the screen. Before the nodes can be used, they have to be connected with the "file reader" node, and with one another by arrows, drawn, again, simply by left clicking the small triangles attached to the nodes. Right clicking on the file reader enables to configure from your computer a requested data file…click Browse…and download from the appropriate folder a csv type Excel file. You are set for analysis now.

Note: the above data file cannot be read by the file reader, and must first be saved as csv type Excel file. For that purpose command in SPSS: click File…click Save as…in "Save as type: enter Comma Delimited (*.csv)…click Save. For your convenience it has been made available in http://extras.springer.com, and entitled "decisiontree".

2.5 Knime Workflow

A knime workflow for the analysis of the above data example is built, and the final result is shown in the underneath figure.

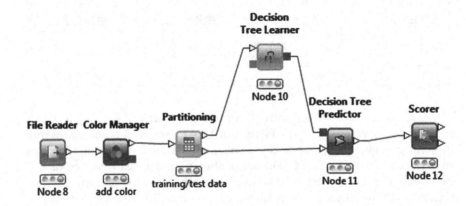

In the node repository click and type color…click the color manager node and drag to workflow editor…in node repository click again color…click the Esc button of your computer…in the node repository click again and type partitioning…the partitioning node is displayed…drag it to the workflow editor…perform the same actions and type respectively Decision Tree Learner, Decision Tree Predictor, and Scorer…Connect, by left clicking, all of the nodes with arrows as indicated above…Configurate and execute all of the nodes by right clicking the nodes and then the texts "Configurate" and "Execute"…the red lights will successively turn orange and then green…right click the Decision Tree Predictor again…right click the text "View: Decision Tree View".

The underneath decision tree comes up. It is pretty much similar to the above SPSS tree, although it does not use 150 cases but only 45 cases (the test sample). Fibrinogen is again the best predictor. A level <29 mg/l gives you 100 % chance of severity score A. A level 29–57.5 gives 92.1 % chance of Severity B, and a level over 57.5 gives 100 % chance of severity C.

Right clicking the scorer node gives you the accuracy statistics, and shows that the sensitivity of A, B, an C are respectively 100, 93.3, and 90.5 %, and that the overall accuracy is 94 %, slightly less than that of the SPSS tree (94.7 %), but still pretty good. In addition, the current analysis is appropriate, and does not use identical data twice.

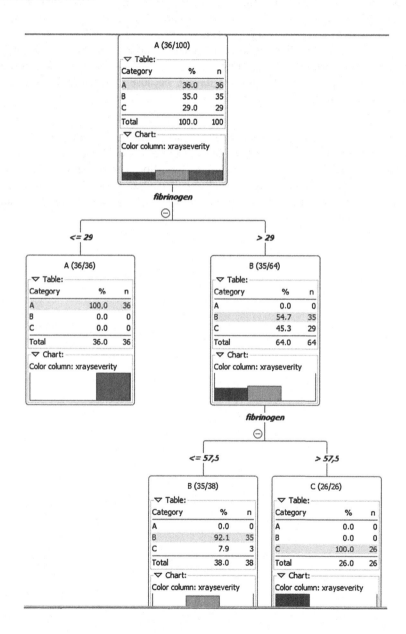

2.6 Conclusion

Traditionally, decision trees are used for finding the best predictors of health risks and improvements. However, this method is not entirely appropriate, because a decision tree is built from a data file, and, subsequently, the same data file is applied once more for computing the health risk probabilities from the built tree. Obviously, the accuracy must be close to 100 %, because the test sample is 100 % identical to the sample used for building the tree, and, therefore, this accuracy does not mean too much. A decision tree with partitioning of a training and a test sample provides similar results, but is scientifically less flawed, because each datum is used only once. In spite of this, little accuracy is lost.

Note
More background, theoretical and mathematical information of decision trees and neural networks are in Machine Learning in Medicine Cookbook One, Chap. 16, pp. 97–104, Decision trees for decision analysis, Springer Heidelberg Germany, 2014, and in Machine Learning in Medicine Part One, Chap. 12, pp. 145–156, Artificial intelligence, multilayer perceptron modeling, Springer Heidelberg Germany, 2013, both by the same authors.

Part II
Linear Models

Chapter 3
Variance Components for Assessing the Magnitude of Random Effects (40 Patients with Paroxysmal Tachycardias)

3.1 General Purpose

If we have reasons to believe that in a study certain patients due to co-morbidity, co-medication and other factors will respond differently from others, then the spread in the data is caused not only by residual effect, but also by some subgroup property, otherwise called some random effect. Variance components analysis is able to assess the magnitudes of random effects as compared to that of the residual error of a study.

3.2 Primary Scientific Question

Can a variance components analysis by including the random effect in the analysis reduce the unexplained variance in a study, and, thus, increase the accuracy of the analysis model as used.

3.3 Example

Variables			
PAT	Treat	Gender	cad
52.00	0.00	0.00	2.00
48.00	0.00	0.00	2.00
43.00	0.00	0.00	1.00
50.00	0.00	0.00	2.00

(continued)

© The Author(s) 2014
T.J. Cleophas and A.H. Zwinderman, *Machine Learning in Medicine—Cookbook Three*, SpringerBriefs in Statistics, DOI 10.1007/978-3-319-12163-5_3

(continued)

Variables			
PAT	Treat	Gender	cad
43.00	0.00	0.00	2.00
44.00	0.00	0.00	1.00
46.00	0.00	0.00	2.00
46.00	0.00	0.00	2.00
43.00	0.00	0.00	1.00
49.00	0.00	0.00	2.00
28.00	1.00	0.00	1.00
35.00	1.00	0.00	2.00

PAT episodes of paroxysmal atrial tachycardias
Treat treatment modality (*0* placebo treatment, *1* active treatment)
Gender gender (*0* female)
cad presence of coronary artery disease (*1* no, *2* yes)

The first 12 of a 40 patient parallel-group study of the treatment of paroxysmal tachycardia with numbers of episodes of PAT as outcome is given above. The entire data file is in "variancecomponents", and is available at http://extras.springer.com. We had reason to believe that the presence of coronary artery disease would affect the outcome, and, therefore, used this variable as a random rather than fixed variable. SPSS statistical software was used for data analysis. Start by opening the data file in SPSS.

Command:
Analyze…General Linear Model…Variance Components…Dependent Variable: enter "paroxtachyc"…Fixed Factor(s): enter "treat, gender"…Random Factor(s): enter "corartdisease"…Model: mark Custom…Model: enter "treat, gender, cad"…click Continue…click Options…mark ANOVA…mark Type III…mark Sums of squares…mark Expected mean squares…click Continue… click OK.

The output sheets are given underneath. The Variance Estimate table gives the magnitude of the Variance due to cad, and that due to residual error (unexplained variance, otherwise called Error). The ratio of the Var(cad)/[Var(Error) + Var(cad)] gives the proportion of variance in the data due to the random cad effect (5.844/ (28.426 + 5.844) = 0.206 = 20.6 %). This means that 79.4 % instead of 100 % of the error is now unexplained.

Variance Estimates

Component	Estimate
Var(cad)	5.844
Var(Error)	28.426

Dependent
Variable: paroxtach
Method: ANOVA
(Type III Sum of
Squares)

The underneath ANOVA table gives the sums of squares and mean squares of different effects. E.g. the mean square of cad = 139.469, and that of residual effect = 28.426.

ANOVA

Source	Type III Sum of Squares	df	Mean Square
Corrected Model	727.069	3	242.356
Intercept	57153.600	1	57153.600
treat	515.403	1	515.403
gender	0.524	1	0.524
cad	139.469	1	139.469
Error	1023.331	36	28.426
Total	58904.000	40	
Corrected Total	1750.400	39	

Dependent Variable: paroxtach

The underneath Expected Mean Squares table gives the results of a special procedure, whereby variances of best fit quadratic functions of the variables are minimized to obtain the best unbiased estimate of the variance components. A little mental arithmetic is now required.

Expected Mean Squares

	Variance Component		
Source	Var(cad)	Var(Error)	Quadratic Term
Intercept	20.000	1.000	Intercept, treat, gender
treat	0.000	1.000	treat
gender	0.000	1.000	gender
cad	19.000	1.000	
Error	0.000	1.000	

Dependent Variable: paroxtach
Expected Mean Squares are based on Type III
Sums of Squares.
For each source, the expected mean square
equals the sum of the coefficients in the cells
times the variance components, plus a
quadratic term involving effects in the
Quadratic Term cell.

EMS (expected mean square) of cad (the random effect)

$= 19 \times$ Variance (cad) $+$ Variance (Error)

$= 139.469$

EMS of Error (the residual effect)

$= 0 +$ Variance (Error)

$= 28.426$

EMS of cad $-$ Variance (Error)

$= 19 \times$ Variance (cad)

$= 139.469 - 28.426$

$= 110.043$

Variance (cad)

$= 110.043/19$

$= 5.844$ (compare with the results of the above Variance Estimates table)

It can, thus, be concluded that around 20 % of the uncertainty is in the data is caused by the random effect.

3.4 Conclusion

If we have reasons to believe that in a study certain patients due to co-morbidity, co-medication and other factors will respond differently from others, then the spread in the data will be caused, not only by the residual effect, but also by the subgroup property, otherwise called the random effect. Variance components analysis, by including the random effect in the analysis, reduces the unexplained variance in a study, and, thus, increases the accuracy of the analysis model used.

Note

More background, theoretical and mathematical information of random effects models are given in Machine Learning in Medicine Part Three, Chap. 9, Random effects, pp. 81–94, 2013, Springer Heidelberg Germany, from the same authors.

Chapter 4
Ordinal Scaling for Clinical Scores with Inconsistent Intervals (900 Patients with Different Levels of Health)

4.1 General Purpose

Clinical studies often have categories as outcome, like various levels of health or disease. Multinomial regression is suitable for analysis (see Chap. 4, Machine Learning in Medicine Cookbook Two, Polynomial regression for outcome categories, pp. 23–25, Springer Heidelberg Germany, 2014, from the same authors). However, if one or two outcome categories in a study are severely underpresented, polynomial regression is flawed, and ordinal regression including specific link functions may provide a better fit for the data.

4.2 Primary Scientific Questions

This chapter is to assess how ordinal regression performs in studies where clinical scores have inconsistent intervals.

4.3 Example

In 900 patients the independent predictors for different degrees of feeling healthy were assessed. The predictors included were:

© The Author(s) 2014
T.J. Cleophas and A.H. Zwinderman, *Machine Learning in Medicine—Cookbook Three*, SpringerBriefs in Statistics, DOI 10.1007/978-3-319-12163-5_4

Variable	2	Fruit consumption (times per week)
	3	Unhealthy snacks (times per week)
	4	Fastfood consumption (times per week)
	5	Physical activities (times per week)
	6	Age (number of years)

Feeling healthy (Variable 1) was assessed as mutually elusive categories:

1. very much so
2. much so
3. not entirely so
4. not so
5. not so at all.

Underneath are the first 10 patients of the data file. The entire data file is in http://extras.springer.com, and is entitled "ordinalscaling".

Variables					
1	2	3	4	5	6
4	6	9	12	6	34
4	7	24	3	6	35
4	3	5	9	6	30
4	5	14	6	3	36
4	9	9	12	12	62
2	2	3	3	6	31
3	3	26	6	3	57
5	9	38	6	6	36
4	5	8	9	6	28
5	9	25	12	12	28

First, we will perform a multinomial regression analysis using SPSS statistical software. Open the data file in SPSS.

Command:
Analyze…Regression…Multinomial Logistic Regression…Dependent: enter feeling healthy…Covariates: enter fruit/week, snacks.week, fastfood/week, physicalactivities/week, age in years…click OK.

Parameter Estimates

feeling healthy[a]		B	Std. Error	Wald	df	Sig.	Exp(B)	95% Confidence Interval for Exp (B)	
								Lower Bound	Upper Bound
very much so	Intercept	−1.252	0.906	1.912	1	0.167			
	fruit	0.149	0.069	4.592	1	0.032	1.161	1.013	1.330
	snacks	0.020	0.017	1.415	1	0.234	1.020	0.987	1.055
	fastfood	−0.079	0.057	1.904	1	0.168	0.924	0.827	1.034
	physical	−0.013	0.056	0.059	1	0.809	0.987	0.885	1.100
	age	−0.027	0.017	2.489	1	0.115	0.974	0.942	1.007
much so	Intercept	−2.087	0.863	5.853	1	0.016			
	fruit	0.108	0.071	2.302	1	0.129	1.114	0.969	1.280
	snacks	−0.001	0.019	0.004	1	0.950	0.999	0.962	1.037
	fastfood	0.026	0.057	0.212	1	0.645	1.026	0.919	1.147
	physical	−0.005	0.051	0.009	1	0.925	0.995	0.900	1.101
	age	−0.010	0.014	0.522	1	0.470	0.990	0.962	1.018
not entirely so	Intercept	2.161	0.418	26.735	1	0.000			
	fruit	0.045	0.039	1.345	1	0.246	1.046	0.969	1.130
	snacks	−0.012	0.011	1.310	1	0.252	0.988	0.968	1.009
	fastfood	−0.037	0.027	1.863	1	0.172	0.964	0.914	1.016
	physical	−0.040	0.025	2.518	1	0.113	0.961	0.914	1.010
	age	−0.028	0.007	14.738	1	0.000	0.972	0.959	0.986
no so	Intercept	0.781	0.529	2.181	1	0.140			
	fruit	0.100	0.046	4.600	1	0.032	1.105	1.009	1.210
	snacks	−0.001	0.012	0.006	1	0.939	0.999	0.975	1.024
	fastfood	−0.038	0.034	1.225	1	0.268	0.963	0.901	1.029
	physical	−0.037	0.032	1.359	1	0.244	0.963	0.905	1.026
	age	−0.028	0.010	8.651	1	0.003	0.972	0.954	0.991

a. The reference category is: not so at all.

The above table gives the analysis results. Twenty-four p-values are produced, and a few of them are statistically significant at $p < 0.05$. For example, per fruit unit you may have 1.161 times more chance of feeling very healthy versus not healthy at all at $p = 0.032$. And per year of age you may have 0.972 times less chance of feeling not entirely healthy versus not healthy at all at $p = 0.0001$. We should add that the few significant p-values among the many insignificant ones could easily be due to type I errors (due to multiple testing). Also a flawed analysis due to inconsistent intervals has not yet been excluded. To assess this point a graph will be drawn.

Command:
Graphs...Legacy Dialogs...Bar...click Simple...mark Summary for groups of cases...click Define...Category Axis: enter "feeling healthy"...click OK.

The underneath graph is in the output sheet. It shows that, particularly the categories 1 and 2 are severely underpresented. Ordinal regression analysis with a complimentary log-log function gives little weight to small counts, and more weight to large counts, and may, therefore, better fit these data.

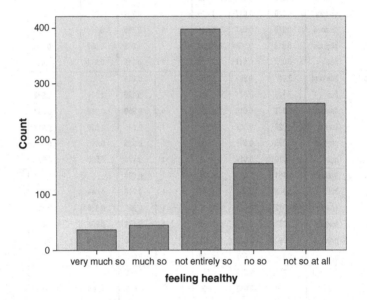

Command:
Analyze...Regression...Ordinal Regression...Dependent: enter feeling healthy... Covariates: enter fruit/week, snacks.week, fastfood/week, physicalactivities/week, age in years...click Options...Link: click Complementary Log-log... click Continue...click OK.

Model Fitting Information

Model	−2 Log Likelihood	Chi-Square	df	Sig.
Intercept Only	2349.631			
Final	2321.863	27.768	5	0.000

Link function: Complementary Log-log.

In the output sheets the model fitting table shows that the ordinal model provides an excellent fit for the data.

Parameter Estimates

		Estimate	Std. Error	Wald	df	Sig.	95% Confidence Interval	
							Lower Bound	Upper Bound
Threshold	[feelinghealthy = 1]	-2.427	0.259	87.865	1	0.000	-2.935	-1.920
	[feelinghealthy = 2]	-1.605	0.229	49.229	1	0.000	-2.053	-1.156
	[feelinghealthy = 3]	0.483	0.208	5.414	1	0.020	0.076	0.890
	[feelinghealthy = 4]	0.971	0.208	21.821	1	0.000	0.564	1.379
Location	fruit	-0.036	0.018	3.907	1	0.048	-0.072	0.000
	snacks	0.004	0.005	0.494	1	0.482	-0.006	0.013
	fastfood	0.017	0.013	1.576	1	0.209	-0.009	0.042
	physical	0.017	0.012	1.772	1	0.183	-0.008	0.041
	age	0.015	0.004	15.393	1	0.000	0.008	0.023

Link function: Complementary Log-log.

The above table is also shown, and indicates that fruit and age are significant predictors of levels of feeling healthy. The less fruit/week, the more chance of feeling healthy versus not healthy at all ($p = 0.048$), the higher the age the more chance of feeling healthy versus not healthy at all ($p = 0.0001$).

4.4 Conclusion

Clinical studies often have categories as outcome, like various levels of health or disease. Multinomial regression is suitable for analysis, but, if one or two outcome categories in a study are severely underpresented, ordinal regression including specific link functions may better fit the data. The current chapter also shows that, unlike multinomial regression, ordinal regression tests the outcome categories as an overall function.

Note
More background, theoretical and mathematical information of multinomial regression is given in Chap. 4, Machine Learning in Medicine Cookbook Two, Polynomial regression for outcome categories, pp. 23–25, Springer Heidelberg Germany, 2014, from the same authors.

Chapter 5
Loglinear Models for Assessing Incident Rates with Varying Incident Risks (12 Populations with Different Drink Consumption Patterns)

5.1 General Purpose

Data files that assess the effect of various predictors on frequency counts of morbidities/mortalities can be classified into multiple cells with varying incident risks (like, e.g., the incident risk of infarction). The underneath table gives an example.

In patients at risk of infarction with little soft drink consumption, and consumption of wine and other alcoholic beverages the incident risk of infarction equals 240/930 = 24.2 %, in those with lots of soft drinks, no wine, and no alcohol otherwise it is 285/1,043 = 27.3 %.

Soft drink (1 = little)	Wine (0 = no)	Alc beverages (0 = no)	Infarcts number	Population number
1.00	1.00	1.00	240	993
1.00	1.00	0.00	237	998
2.00	1.00	1.00	236	1,016
2.00	1.00	0.00	236	1,011
3.00	1.00	1.00	221	1,004
3.00	1.00	0.00	221	1,003
1.00	0.00	1.00	270	939

(continued)

© The Author(s) 2014
T.J. Cleophas and A.H. Zwinderman, *Machine Learning in Medicine—Cookbook Three*, SpringerBriefs in Statistics, DOI 10.1007/978-3-319-12163-5_5

(continued)

Soft drink (1 = little)	Wine (0 = no)	Alc beverages (0 = no)	Infarcts number	Population number
1.00	0.00	0.00	269	940
2.00	0.00	1.00	274	979
2.00	0.00	0.00	273	966
3.00	0.00	1.00	284	1,041
3.00	0.00	0.00	285	1,043

The general loglinear model using Poisson distributions (see Statistics Applied to Clinical Studies 5th Edition, Chap. 23, Poisson regression, pp. 267–275, Springer Heidelberg Germany, 2012, from the same authors) is an appropriate method for statistical testing. This chapter is to assess this method, frequently used by banks and insurance companies but little by clinicians so far.

5.2 Primary Scientific Question

Can general loglinear modeling identify subgroups with significantly larger incident risks than other subgroups.

5.3 Example

The example in the above table will be applied. We wish to investigate the effect of soft drink, wine, and other alcoholic beverages on the risk of infarction. The data file is in http://extras.springer.com, and is entitled "loglinear". Start by opening the file in SPSS statistical software.

> Command:
> Analyze...Loglinear...General Loglinear Analysis...Factor(s): enter softdrink, wine, other alc beverages...click "Data" in the upper text row of your screen... click Weigh Cases...mark Weight cases by...Frequency Variable: enter "infarcts"...click OK...return to General Loglinear Analysis...Cell structure: enter "population"... Options ...mark Estimates...click Continue...Distribution of Cell Counts: mark Poisson...click OK.

The above pretty dull table gives some wonderful information. The soft drink classes 1 and 2 are not significantly different from zero. These classes have, thus, no greater risk of infarction than class 3. However, the regression coefficient of no wine is greater than zero at $p = 0.016$. No wine drinkers have a significantly greater

Parameter Estimates[b,c]

Parameter	Estimate	Std. Error	Z	Sig.	95% Confidence Interval	
					Lower Bound	Upper Bound
Constant	1.513	0.067	−22.496	0.000	−1,645	−1.381
[softdrink = 1.00]	0.095	0.093	1.021	0.307	−0.088	0.278
[softdrink = 2.00]	0.053	0.094	0.569	0.569	−0.130	0.237
[softdrink = 3.00]	0[a]	.	.	.	.	.
[wine = 0.00]	0.215	0.090	2.403	0.016	0.040	0.391
[wine = 1.00]	0[a]	.	.	.	.	.
[alcbeverages = 0.00]	0.003	0.095	0.029	0.977	−0.184	0.189
[alcbeverages = 1.00]	0[a]	.	.	.	.	.
[softdrink = 1.00] * [wine = 0.00]	−0.043	0.126	−0.345	0.730	−0.291	0.204
[softdrink = 1.00] * [wine = 1.00]	0[a]	.	.	.	.	.
[softdrink = 2.00] * [wine = 0.00]	−0.026	0.126	−0.209	0.834	−0.274	0.221
[softdrink = 2.00] * [wine = 1.00]	0[a]	.	.	.	.	.
[softdrink = 3.00] * [wine = 0.00]	0[a]	.	.	.	.	.
[softdrink = 3.00] * [wine = 1.00]	0[a]	.	.	.	.	.
[softdrink = 1.00] * [alcbeverages = 0.00]	−0.021	0.132	−0.161	0.872	−0.280	0.237
[softdrink = 1.00] * [alcbeverages = 1.00]	0[a]	.	.	.	.	.
[softdrink = 2.00] * [alcbeverages =0.00]	0.003	0.132	0.024	0.981	−0.256	0.262
[softdrink = 2.00] * [alcbeverages = 1.00]	0[a]	.	.	.	.	.
[softdrink = 3.00] * [alcbeverages = 0.00]	0[a]	.	.	.	.	.
[softdrink = 3.00] * [alcbeverages = 1.00]	0[a]	.	.	.	.	.
[wine = 0.00] * [alcbeverages = 0.00]	−0.002	0.127	−0.018	0.986	−0.251	0.246
[wine = 0.00] * [alcbeverages = 1.00]	0[a]	.	.	.	.	.
[wine = 1.00] * [alcbeverages = 0.00]	0[a]	.	.	.	.	.
[wine = 1.00] * [alcbeverages = 1.00]	0[a]	.	.	.	.	.
[softdrink = 1.00] * [wine = 0.00] * [alcbeverages =0.00]	0.016	0.178	0.089	0.929	−0.334	0.366
[softdrink = 1.00] * [wine = 0.00] * [alcbeverages = 1.00]	0[a]	.	.	.	.	.
[softdrink = 1.00] * [wine = 1.00] * [alcbeverages = 0.00]	0[a]	.	.	.	.	.
[softdrink = 1.00] * [wine = 1.00] * [alcbeverages = 1.00]	0[a]	.	.	.	.	.
[softdrink = 2.00] * [wine =0.00] * [alcbeverages = 0.00]	0.006	0.178	0.036	0.971	−0.343	0.356
[softdrink = 2,00] * [wine =0.00] * [alcbeverages = 1.00]	0[a]	.	.	.	.	.
[softdrink = 2.00] * [wine = 1.00] * [alcbeverages = 0.00]	0[a]	.	.	.	.	.
[softdrink = 2.00] * [wine = 1.00] * [alcbeverages = 1.00]	0[a]	.	.	.	.	.
[softdrink = 3.00] * [wine =0.00] * [alcbeverages = 0.00]	0[a]	.	.	.	.	.
[softdrink = 3,00] * [wine =0.00] * [alcbeverages = 1.00]	0[a]	.	.	.	.	.
[softdrink = 3,00] * [wine = 1.00] * [alcbeverages =0.00]	0[a]	.	.	.	.	.
[softdrink = 3.00] * [wine = 1.00] * [alcbeverages = 1.00]	0[a]	.	.	.	.	.

a. This parameter is set to zero because it is redundant.
b. Model: Poisson
c. Design: Constant + softdrink + wine + alcbeverages + softdrink * wine + softdrink * alcbeverages + wine * alcbeverages + softdrink * wine * alcbeverages

risk of infarction than the wine drinkers have. No "other alcoholic beverages" did not protect from infarction better than the consumption of it. The three predictors did not display any interaction effects. This result would be in agreement with the famous French paradox.

5.4 Conclusion

Data files that assess the effect of various predictors on frequency counts of morbidities/mortalities can be classified into multiple cells with varying incident risks (like, e.g., the incident risk of infarction). The general loglinear model using Poisson distributions is an appropriate method for statistical testing. It can identify subgroups with significantly larger incident risks than other subgroups.

Note
More background, theoretical and mathematical information of Poisson regression is given in Statistics Applied to Clinical Studies 5th Edition, Chap. 23, Poisson regression, pp. 267–275, Springer Heidelberg Germany, 2012, from the same authors.

Chapter 6
Loglinear Modeling for Outcome Categories (Quality of Life Scores in 445 Patients with Different Personal Characteristics)

6.1 General Purpose

Multinomial regression is adequate for identifying the main predictors of certain outcome categories, like different levels of injury or quality of life (QOL) (see Machine Learning in Medicine Cookbook Two, Chap. 4, pp. 23–25, Polynomial regression for outcome categories, 2014, Springer Heidelberg Germany, from the same authors). An alternative approach is logit loglinear modeling. The latter method does not use continuous predictors on a case by case basis, but rather the weighted means of these predictors. This approach may allow for relevant additional conclusions from your data.

6.2 Primary Scientific Question

Does logit loglinear modeling allow for relevant additional conclusions from your categorical data as compared to polynomial/multinomial regression?

6.3 Example

Age	Gender	Married	Lifestyle	qol
55	1	0	0	2
32	1	1	1	2
27	1	1	0	1
77	0	1	0	3
34	1	1	0	1

(continued)

© The Author(s) 2014
T.J. Cleophas and A.H. Zwinderman, *Machine Learning in Medicine—Cookbook Three*, SpringerBriefs in Statistics,
DOI 10.1007/978-3-319-12163-5_6

(continued)

Age	Gender	Married	Lifestyle	qol
35	1	0	1	1
57	1	1	1	2
57	1	1	1	2
35	0	0	0	1
42	1	1	0	2
30	0	1	0	3
34	0	1	1	1

Variable
1. *Age* (years)
2. *Gender* (*0* female)
3. *Married* (*0* no)
4. *Lifestyle* (*0* poor)
5. *qol* (quality of life levels *0* low, *2* high)

The above table show the data of the first 12 patients of a 445 patient data file of qol (quality of life) levels and patient characteristics. The characteristics are the predictor variables of the qol levels (the outcome variable). The entire data file is in http://extras.springer.com, and is entitled "logitloglinear". We will first perform a traditional polynomial regression and then the logit loglinear model. SPSS statistical is used for analysis. Start by opening SPSS, and entering the data file.

Command:
Analyze...Regression...Multinomial Logistic Regression...Dependent: enter "qol"...Factor(s): enter "gender, married, lifestyle"...Covariate(s): enter "age"...OK.

The underneath table shows the main results. The following conclusions are appropriate.

Parameter Estimates

qol[a]		B	Std. Error	Wald	df	Sig.	Exp(B)	95% Confidence Interval for Exp (B) Lower Bound	Upper Bound
low	Intercept	28.027	2.539	121.826	1	0.000			
	age	−0.559	0.047	143.158	1	0.000	0.572	0.522	0.626
	[gender=0]	0.080	0.508	0.025	1	0.875	1.083	0.400	2.930
	[gender=1]	0[b]	.	.	0	.	.	.	.
	[married=0]	2.081	0.541	14.784	1	0.000	8.011	2.774	23.140
	[married=1]	0[b]	.	.	0	.	.	.	.
	[lifestyle=0]	−0.801	0.513	2.432	1	0.119	0.449	0.164	1.228
	[lifestyle=1]	0[b]	.	.	0	.	.	.	.
medium	Intercept	20.133	2.329	74.743	1	0.000			
	age	−0.355	0.040	79.904	1	0.000	0.701	0.649	0.758
	[gender=0]	0.306	0.372	0.674	1	0.412	1.358	0.654	2.817
	[gender=1]	0[b]	.	.	0	.	.	.	.
	[married=0]	0.612	0.394	2.406	1	0.121	1.843	0.851	3.992
	[married=1]	0[b]	.	.	0	.	.	.	.
	[lifestyle=0]	−0.014	0.382	0.001	1	0.972	0.987	0.466	2.088
	[lifestyle=1]	0[b]	.	.	0	.	.	.	.

a. The reference category is: high.
b. This parameter is set to zero because it is redundant.

1. The unmarried subjects have a greater chance of QOL level 0 than the married ones (the b-value is positive here).
2. The higher the age, the less chance of QOL levels 0 and 1 (the b-values are negative here). If you wish, you may also report the odds ratios (Exp (B)).

We will now perform a logit loglinear analysis.

Command:
Analyze...Loglinear...Logit...Dependent: enter "qol"...Factor(s): enter "gender, married, lifestyle"...Cell Covariate(s): enter: "age"...Model: Terms in Model: enter: "gender, married, lifestyle, age"...click Continue...click Options...mark Estimates...mark Adjusted residuals...mark normal probabilities for adjusted residuals...click Continue...click OK.

The underneath table shows the observed frequencies per cell, and the frequencies to be expected, if the predictors had no effect on the outcome.

Cell Counts and Residuals[a,b]

				Observed		Expected					
gender	married	lifestyle	qol	Count	%	Count	%	Residual	Standardized Residual	Adjusted Residual	Deviance
Male	Unmarried	Inactive	low	7	23.3%	9.111	30.4%	−2.111	−0.838	−1.125	−1.921
			medium	16	53.3%	14.124	47.1%	1.876	0.686	0.888	1.998
			high	7	23.3%	6.765	22.6%	0.235	0.103	0.127	0.691
		Active	low	29	61.7%	25.840	55.0%	3.160	0.927	2.018	2.587
			medium	5	10.6%	10.087	21.5%	−5.087	−1.807	−2.933	−2.649
			high	13	27.7%	11.074	23.6%	1.926	0.662	2.019	2.042
	Married	Inactive	low	9	11.0%	10.636	13.0%	−1.636	−0.538	−0.826	−1.734
			medium	41	50.0%	43.454	53.0%	−2.454	−0.543	−1.062	−2.183
			high	32	39.0%	27.910	34.0%	4.090	0.953	2.006	2.958
		Active	low	15	23.8%	14.413	22.9%	0.587	0.176	0.754	1.094
			medium	27	42.9%	21.336	33.9%	5.664	1.508	2.761	3.566
			high	21	33.3%	27.251	43.3%	−6.251	−1.590	−2.868	−3.308
Female	Unmarried	Inactive	low	12	26.1%	11.119	24.2%	0.881	0.303	0.627	1.353
			medium	26	56.5%	22.991	50.0%	3.009	0.887	1.601	2.529
			high	8	17.4%	11.890	25.8%	−3.890	−1.310	−1.994	−2.518
		Active	low	18	54.5%	19.930	60.4%	−1.930	−0.687	−0.978	−1.915
			medium	6	18.2%	5.799	17.6%	0.201	0.092	0.138	0.639
			high	9	27.3%	7.271	22.0%	1.729	0.726	1.064	1.959
	Married	Inactive	low	15	18.5%	12.134	15.0%	2.866	0.892	1.670	2.522
			medium	27	33.3%	29.432	36.3%	−2.432	−0.562	−1.781	−2.158
			high	39	48.1%	39.434	48.7%	−0.434	−0.097	−0.358	−0.929
		Active	low	16	25.4%	17.817	28.3%	−1.817	−0.508	−1.123	−1.855
			medium	24	38.1%	24.779	39.3%	−0.779	−0.201	−0.882	−1.238
			high	23	36.5%	20.404	32.4%	2.596	0.699	1.407	2.347

a. Model: Multinomial Logit
b. Design: Constant + qol + qol * gender + qol * married + qol * lifestyle + qol * age

The two graphs below show the goodnesses of fit of the model, which are obviously pretty good, as both expected versus observed counts (first graph below) and q-q plot (second graph below) show excellent linear relationships.

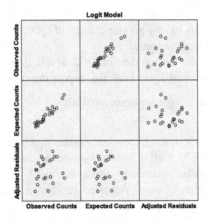

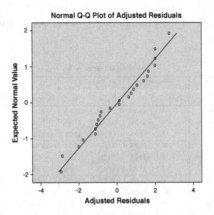

Note: the Q-Q plot (Q stands for quantile) shows here that the differences between observed and expected counts follow a normal distribution.

The next page table shows the results of the statistical tests of the data.

1. The unmarried subjects have a greater chance of QOL 1 (low QOL) than their married counterparts.
2. The poor lifestyle subjects have a greater chance of QOL 1 (low QOL) than their adequate-lifestyle counterparts.
3. The higher the age the more chance of QOL 2 (medium level QOL), which is neither very good nor very bad, nut rather in between (as you would expect).

We may conclude that the two procedures produce similar results, but the latter method provides some additional and relevant information about the lifestyle and age data.

Parameter Estimates[c] [d]

Parameter		Estimate	Std. Error	Z	Sig.	95% Confidence Interval	
						Lower Bound	Upper Bound
Constant	[gender = 0] * [married = 0] * [lifestyle = 0]	−7.402[a]					
	[gender = 0] * [married = 0] * [lifestyle = 1]	−7.409[a]					
	[gender = 0] * [married = 1] * [lifestyle = 0]	−6.088[a]					
	[gender = 0] * [married = 1] * [lifestyle = 1]	−6.349[a]					
	[gender = 1] * [married = 0] * [lifestyle = 0]	−6.825[a]					
	[gender = 1] * [married = 0] * [lifestyle = 1]	−7.406[a]					
	[gender = 1] * [married = 1] * [lifestyle = 0]	−5.960[a]					
	[gender = 1] * [married = 1] * [lifestyle = 1]	−6.567[a]					
[qol = 1]		5.332	8.845	0.603	0.547	−12.004	22.667
[qol = 2]		4.280	10.073	0.425	0.671	−15.463	24.022
[qol = 3]		0[b]	.	.	.	.	.
[qol = 1] * [gender = 0]		0.389	0.360	1.079	0.280	−0.317	1.095
[qol = 1] * [gender = 1]		0[b]	.	.	.	.	.
[qol = 2] * [gender = 0]		−0.140	0.265	−0.528	0.597	660	0.380
[qol = 2] * [gender = 1]		0[b]	.	.	.	.	.
[qol = 3] * [gender = 0]		0[b]	.	.	.	.	.
[qol = 3] * [gender = 1]		0[b]	.	.	.	.	.
[qol = 1] * [married = 0]		1.132	0.283	4.001	0.000	0.578	1.687
[qol = 1] * [married = 1]		0[b]	.	.	.	.	.
[qol = 2] * [married = 0]		−0.078	0.294	−0.267	0.790	−0.655	0.498
[qol = 2] * [married = 1]		0[b]	.	.	.	.	.
[qol = 3] * [married = 0]		0[b]	.	.	.	.	.
[qol = 3] * [married = 1]		0[b]	.	.	.	.	.
[qol = 1] * [lifestyle = 0]		−1.004	0.311	−3.229	0.001	−1.613	−0.394
[qol = 1] * [lifestyle = 1]		0[b]	.	.	.	.	.
[qol = 2] * [lifestyle = 0]		0.016	0.271	0.059	0.953	−0.515	0.547
[qol = 2] * [lifestyle = 1]		0[b]	.	.	.	.	.
[qol = 3] * [lifestyle = 0]		0[b]	.	.	.	.	.
[qol = 3] * [lifestyle = 1]		0[b]	.	.	.	.	.
[qol = 1] * age		0.116	0.074	1.561	0.119	−0.030	0.261
[qol = 2] * age		0.114	0.054	2.115	0.034	0.008	0.219
[qol = 3] * age		0.149	0.138	1.075	0.282	−0.122	0.419

a. Constants are not parameters under the multinomial assumption. Therefore, their standard errors are not calculated.
b. This parameter is set to zero because it is redundant.
c. Model: Multinomial Logit
d. Design: Constant + qol + qol * gender + qol * married + qol * lifestyle + qol * age

6.4 Conclusion

Multinomial regression is adequate for identifying the main predictors of certain outcome categories, like different levels of injury or quality of life. An alternative approach is logit loglinear modeling. The latter method does not use continuous predictors on a case by case basis, but rather the weighted means. This approach allowed for relevant additional conclusions in the example given.

Note

More background, theoretical and mathematical information of polynomial/multinomial regression is given in Machine Learning in Medicine Cookbook Two, Chap. 4, Polynomial regression for outcome categories, pp. 23–25, 2014, Springer Heidelberg Germany, from the same authors. More information of loglinear modeling is in the current volume, Chap. 5, Loglinear models for assessing incident rates with varying incident risks.

Chapter 7
Heterogeneity in Clinical Research: Mechanisms Responsible

7.1 General Purpose

In clinical research similar studies often have different results. This may be due to differences in patient-characteristics and trial-quality-characteristics such as the use of blinding, randomization, and placebo-controls. This chapter is to assess whether 3-dimensional scatter plots and regression analyses with the treatment results as outcome and the predictors of heterogeneity as exposure are able to identify mechanisms responsible.

7.2 Primary Scientific Question

Are scatter plots and regression models able to identify the mechanisms responsible for heterogeneity in clinical research.

7.3 Example

Variables			
1	2	3	4
% ADEs	Study size	Age	Investigator type
21.00	106	1	1
14.40	578	1	1
30.40	240	1	1
6.10	671	0	0
12.00	681	0	0

(continued)

© The Author(s) 2014
T.J. Cleophas and A.H. Zwinderman, *Machine Learning in Medicine—Cookbook Three*, SpringerBriefs in Statistics, DOI 10.1007/978-3-319-12163-5_7

(continued)

Variables			
1	2	3	4
% ADEs	Study size	Age	Investigator type
3.40	28,411	1	0
6.60	347	0	0
3.30	8,601	0	0
4.90	915	0	0
9.60	156	0	0
6.50	4,093	0	0
6.50	18,820	0	0
4.10	6,383	0	0
4.30	2,933	0	0
3.50	480	0	0
4.30	19,070	1	0
12.60	2,169	1	0
33.20	2,261	0	1
5.60	12,793	0	0
5.10	355	0	0

ADEs adverse drug effects
Age *0* young, *1* elderly
Investigator type *0* pharmacists, *1* clinicians

In the above 20 studies the percentage of admissions to hospital due to adverse drug effects were assessed. The studies were very heterogeneous, because the percentages admissions due to adverse drug effects varied from 3.3 to 33.2. In order to identify possible mechanisms responsible, a scatter plot was first drawn. The data file is in http://extras.springer.com and is entitled "heterogeneity".

Start by opening the data file in SPSS statistical software.

Command:
click Graphs...click Legacy Dialogs...click Scatter/Dot...click 3-D Scatter... click Define...Y-Axis: enter percentage (ADEs)...X Axis: enter study-magnitude...Z Axis: enter clinicians = 1...Set Markers by: enter elderly = 1...click OK.

The underneath figure is displayed, and it gives a 3-dimensional graph of the outcome (percentage adverse drug effects) versus study size versus investigator type (1 = clinician, 0 = pharmacist). A 4th dimension is obtained by coloring the circles (green = elderly, blue = young). Small studies tended to have larger results. Also clinician studies (clinicians = 1) tended to have larger results, while studies in elderly had both large and small effects.

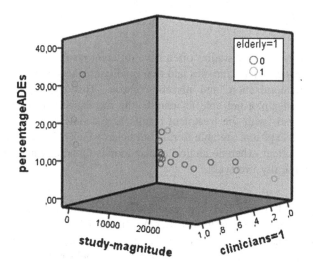

In order to test whether the observed trends were statistically significant, a linear regression is performed.

Command:
Analyze...Regression...Linear...Dependent: enter "percentage ADEs"...Independent(s): enter "study-magnitude, elderly = 1, clinicians = 1"...click OK.

Coefficients[a]

Model		Unstandardized Coefficients		Standardized Coefficients	t	Sig.
		B	Std. Error	Beta		
1	(Constant)	6.924	1.454		4.762	0.000
	study-magnitude	-7.674E-5	0.000	-0.071	-0.500	0.624
	elderly=1	-1.393	2.885	-0.075	-0.483	0.636
	clinicians=1	18.932	3.359	0.887	5.636	0.000

a. Dependent Variable: percentageADEs

The output sheets show the above table. The investigator type is the only statistically significant predictor of percentage of ADEs. Clinicians observed significantly more ADE admissions than did pharmacists at $p < 0.0001$. This is in agreement with the above graph.

7.4 Conclusion

In clinical research similar studies often have different results. This may be due to differences in patient-characteristics and trial-quality-characteristics such as the use of blinding, randomization, and placebo-controls. This chapter shows that 3-dimensional scatter plot are able to identify the mechanisms responsible. Linear regression analyses with the treatment results as outcome and the predictors of heterogeneity as exposure are able to rule out heterogeneity due to chance. This is particularly important, when no clinical explanation is found or when heterogeneity seems to be clinically irrelevant.

Note
More background, theoretical and mathematical information of heterogeneous studies and meta-regression is in Statistics Applied to Clinical Studies 5th Edition, Chap. 33, Meta-analysis, review and update of methodologies, pp. 379–390, and Chap. 34, Meta-regression, pp. 391–397, Springer Heidelberg Germany, both from the same authors as the current work.

Chapter 8
Performance Evaluation of Novel Diagnostic Tests (650 and 588 Patients with Peripheral Vascular Disease)

8.1 General Purpose

Both logistic regression and c-statistics can be used to evaluate the performance of novel diagnostic tests. This chapter is to assess whether one method can outperform the other.

8.2 Primary Scientific Question

Is logistic regression with the odds of disease as outcome and test scores as covariate a better alternative for concordance (c)-statistics using the area under the curve of receiver operated characteristic (ROC) curves.

8.3 Example

In 650 patients with peripheral vascular disease a noninvasive vascular lab test was performed. The results of the first 10 patients are underneath.

© The Author(s) 2014
T.J. Cleophas and A.H. Zwinderman, *Machine Learning in Medicine—Cookbook Three*, SpringerBriefs in Statistics, DOI 10.1007/978-3-319-12163-5_8

Test score	Presence of peripheral vascular disease (0 = no, 1 = yes)
1.00	0.00
1.00	0.00
2.00	0.00
2.00	0.00
3.00	0.00
3.00	0.00
3.00	0.00
4.00	0.00
4.00	0.00
4.00	0.00

The entire data file is in http://extras.springer.com, and is entitled "vascdisease1". Start by opening the data file in SPSS.

Then command:
Graphs...Legacy Dialogs...Histogram...Variable(s): enter "score"...Row(s): enter "disease"...click OK.

The underneath figure shows the output sheet. On the x-axis we have the vascular lab scores, on the y-axis "how often". The scores in patients with (1) and without (0) the presence of disease according to the gold standard (angiography) are respectively in the lower and upper graph.

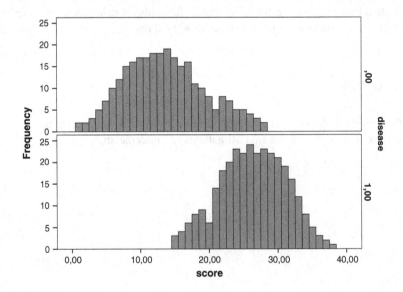

The second data file is obtained from a parallel-group population of 588 patients after the noninvasive vascular test has been improved. The first 10 patients are underneath.

Test score	Presence of peripheral vascular disease (0 = no, 1 = yes)
1.00	0.00
2.00	0.00
2.00	0.00
3.00	0.00
3.00	0.00
3.00	0.00
4.00	0.00
4.00	0.00
4.00	0.00
4.00	0.00

The entire data file is in http://extras.springer.com, and is entitled "vascdisease2". Start by opening the data file in SPSS.

Then command:
Graphs...Legacy Dialogs...Histogram...Variable(s): enter "score"...Row(s): enter "disease"...click OK.

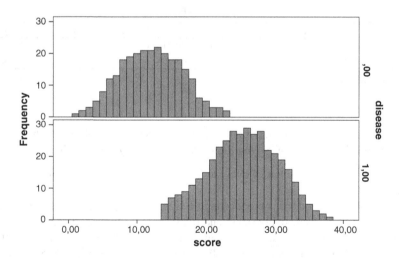

The above figure is in the output sheet.

The first test (upper figure) seems to perform less well than the second test (lower figure), because there may be more risk of false positives (the 0 disease curve is more skewed to the right in the upper than in the lower figure).

8.3.1 Binary Logistic Regression

Binary logistic regression is used for assessing this question. The following rea-
soning is used. If we move the threshold for a positive test to the right, then the
proportion of false positive will decrease. The steeper the logistic regression line the
faster this will happen. In contrast, if we move the threshold to the left, the proportion of false negatives will decrease. Again, the steeper the logistic regression
line, the faster it will happen. And so, the steeper the logistic regression line, the
fewer false negatives and false positives and thus the better the diagnostic test.
   For both data files the above analysis is performed.

   Command:
   Analyze...Regression...Binary logistic...Dependent variable: disease...Covar-
iate: score...OK.

   The output sheets show the best fit regression equations.

Variables in the Equation

		B	S.E.	Wald	df	Sig.	Exp(B)
Step 1[a]	VAR00001	0.398	0.032	155.804	1	0.000	1.488
	Constant	−8.003	0.671	142.414	1	0.000	0.000

a. Variable(s) entered on step 1: VAR00001.

Variables in the Equation

		B	S.E.	Wald	df	Sig.	Exp(B)
Step 1[a]	VAR00001	0.581	0.051	130.715	1	0.000	1.789
	Constant	−10.297	0.915	126.604	1	0.000	0.000

a. Variable(s) entered on step 1: VAR00001.

   Data file 1: log odds of having the disease = −8.003 + 0.398 times the score
   Data file 2: log odds of having the disease = −10.297 + 0.581 times the score.

   The regression coefficient of data file 2 is much steeper than that of data file 1,
0.581 and 0.398.
   Both regression equations produce highly significant regression coefficients with
standard errors of respectively 0.032 and 0.051 and p-values of <0.0001. The two
regression coefficients are tested for significance of difference using the z-test (the
z-test is in Chap. 2 of Statistics on a Pocket Calculator part 2, pp. 3–5, Springer
Heidelberg Germany, 2012, from the same authors):

$$z = (0.398 - 0.581)/\sqrt{(0.032^2 + 0.051^2)} = -0.183/0.060 = -3.05,$$

which corresponds with a p-value of <0.01.

Obviously, test 2 produces a significantly steeper regression model, which means that it is a better predictor of the risk of disease than test 1. We can, additionally, calculate the odds ratios of successfully testing with test 2 versus test 1. The odds of disease with test 1 equals $e^{0.398} = 1.488$, and with test 2 it equals $e^{0.581} = 1.789$. The odds ratio $= 1.789/1.488 = 1.202$, meaning that the second test produces a 1.202 times better chance of rightly predicting the disease than test 1 does.

8.3.2 c-Statistics

c-Statistics is used as a contrast test. Open data file 1 again.

Command:
Analyze...ROC Curve...Test Variable: enter "score"...State Variable: enter "disease"...Value of State Variable: type "1"...mark ROC Curve...mark Standard Error and Confidence Intervals...click OK.

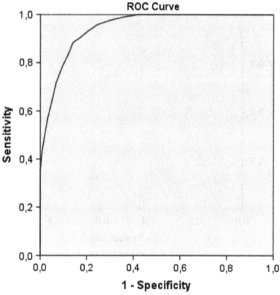

Diagonal segments are produced by ties.

Area Under the Curve

Test Result Variable(s):score

			Asymptotic 95% Confidence Interval	
Area	Std. Error[a]	Asymptotic Sig.[b]	Lower Bound	Upper Bound
0.945	0.009	0.000	0.928	0.961

The test result variable(s): score has at least one tie between the positive actual state group and the negative actual state group. Statistics may be biased.

a. Under the nonparametric assumption
b. Null hypothesis: true area = 0.5

Subsequently the same procedure is followed for data file 2.

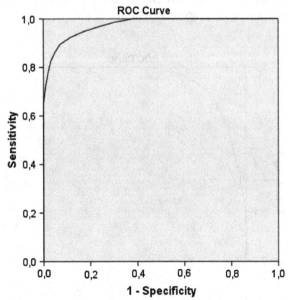

ROC Curve

1 - Specificity

Diagonal segments are produced by ties.

!

The Area under curve of data file 2 is larger than that of data file 1. The test 2 seems to perform better. The z-test can again be used to test for significance of difference.

$$z = (0.974 - 0.945)/\sqrt{(0.009^2 + 0.005^2)} = 2.90$$
$$p = <0.01.1.$$

Area Under the Curve

Test Result Variable(s):score

			Asymptotic 95% Confidence Interval	
Area	Std. Error[a]	Asymptotic Sig.[b]	Lower Bound	Upper Bound
0.974	0.005	0.000	0.965	0.983

The test result variable(s): score has at least one tie between the positive actual state group and the negative actual state group. Statistics may be biased.

a. Under the nonparametric assumption
b. Null hypothesis: true area = 0.5

8.4 Conclusion

Both logistic regression with the presence of disease as outcome and test scores of as predictor and c-statistics can be used for comparing the performance of qualitative diagnostic tests. However, c-statistics may perform less well with very large areas under the curve, and it assesses relative risks while in practice absolute risk levels may be more important.

Note

More background, theoretical and mathematical information of logistic regression and c-statistics is in Machine Learning in Medicine Part Two, Chap. 6, pp. 45–52, Logistics regression for assessment of novel diagnostic tests against controls, Springer Heidelberg Germany, 2013, from the same authors.

Part III
Rules Models

Chapter 9
Spectral Plots for High Sensitivity Assessment of Periodicity (6 Years' Monthly C Reactive Protein Levels)

9.1 General Purpose

In clinical research times series often show many peaks and irregular spaces.

Spectral plots is based on traditional Fourier analyses, and may be more sensitive than traditional autocorrelation analysis in this situation.

9.2 Specific Scientific Question

To assess whether, in monthly C reactive Protein (CRP) levels with inconclusive scattergrams and autocorrelation analysis, spectral plot methodology is able to demonstrate periodicity even so.

9.3 Example

A data file of 6 years' mean monthly CRP levels from a target population was assessed for seasonality. The first 2 years' values are given underneath. The entire data file is in "spectralanalysis" as available on the internet at http://extras.springer.com.

First day of month	CRP level (mg/l)
1993/07/01	1.29
1993/08/01	1.43
1993/09/01	1.54
1993/10/01	1.68

(continued)

© The Author(s) 2014
T.J. Cleophas and A.H. Zwinderman, *Machine Learning in Medicine—Cookbook Three*, SpringerBriefs in Statistics, DOI 10.1007/978-3-319-12163-5_9

(continued)

First day of month	CRP level (mg/l)
1993/11/01	1.54
1993/12/01	2.78
1994/01/01	1.27
1994/02/01	1.26
1994/03/01	1.26
1994/04/01	1.54
1994/05/01	1.13
1994/06/01	1.60
1994/07/01	1.47
1994/08/01	1.78
1994/09/01	2.69
1994/10/01	1.91
1994/11/01	1.74
1994/12/01	3.11

Start by opening the data file in SPSS.

Command:
Click Graphs...click Legacy Dialogs...click Scatter/Dot... Click Simple Scatter...click Define...y-axis: enter "mean crp mg/l"...x-axis: enter date...click OK.

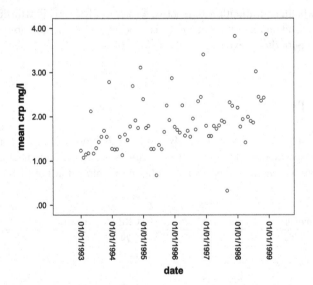

In the output the above figure is displayed. Many peaks and irregularities are observed, and the presence of periodicity is not unequivocal.

Subsequently, autocorrelation coefficients are computed.

Command:
click Analyze...click Forecast...click Autocorrelations...Variables: enter "mean crp mg/l"...click OK.

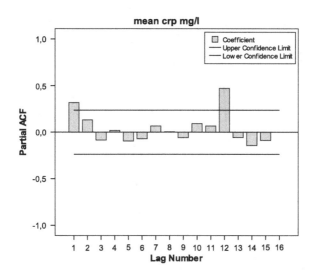

In the output the above autocorrelation coefficients are given. It suggests the presence of periodicity. However, this conclusion is based on a single value, i.e., the 12th month value, and, for concluding unequivocal periodicity not only autocorrelation coefficients significantly larger than 0 but also significantly smaller than 0 should have been observed.

Spectral plots may be helpful for support.

Command:
Analyze...Forecasting...Spectral Analysis...select CRP and enter into Variable (s)...select Spectral density in Plot...click Paste...change in syntax text: TSET PRINT-DEFAULT into TSET PRINT-DETAILED... click Run...click All.

In the output sheets underneath the *periodogram* is observed (upper part) with mean CRP values on the y-axis and frequencies on the x-axis. Of the peaks CRP-values observed the first one has a frequency of slightly less than 0.1. We assumed that CRP had an annual periodicity. Twelve months are in a year, months is the unit applied. As period is the inverted value of frequency a period of 12 months would equal a frequency of $1/12 = 0.0833$. An annual periodicity would produce a peak

CRP-value with a frequency of 1/12 = 0.0833. Indeed, the table underneath shows that at a frequency of 0.0833 the highest CRP value is observed. However, many more peaks are observed, and how to interpret them. For that purpose we use *spectral density analysis* (lower figure underneath).

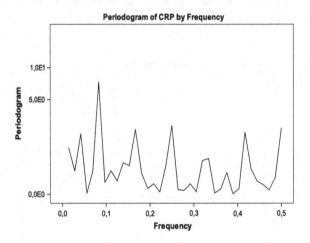

Periodogram of CRP by Frequency

Univariate Statistics

Series Name:mean crp mg/l

	Frequency	Period	Sine Transform	Cosine Transform	Periodogram	Spectral Density Estimate
1	0.00000		0.000	1.852	0.000	8.767
2	0.01389		−0.197	0.020	1.416	12.285
3	0.02778		−0.123	0.012	0.552	9.223
4	0.04167		−0.231	0.078	2.144	10.429
5	0.05556		0.019	0.010	0.016	23.564
6	0.06944		−0.040	−0.117	0.552	22.985
7	0.08333		−0.365	0.267	7.355	19.519
8	0.09722		−0.057	−0.060	0.243	20.068
9	0.11111		−0.101	−0.072	0.556	20.505
10	0.12500		−0.004	−0.089	0.286	5.815
11	0.13889		0.065	−0.135	0.811	10.653
12	0.15278		−0.024	0.139	0.715	10.559

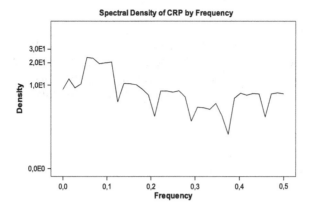

The spectral density curve is a filtered, otherwise called smoothed, version of the usual periodogram with irregularities beyond a given threshold (noise) filtered out. The above spectral density curve shows five distinct peaks with a rather regular pattern. The lowest frequency simply displays the yearly peak at a frequency of 0.0833. The other peaks at higher frequencies are the result of the Fourier model consistent of sine and cosine functions, and do not indicate additional periodicities. Even so much so that they demonstrate the absence of further periodicities.

9.4 Conclusion

Seasonal patterns are assumed in many fields of medicine. Usually, the mean differences between the data of different seasons or months are used. E.g., the number of hospital admissions in the month of January may be roughly twice that of July. However, biological processes are full of variations and the possibility of chance findings can not be fully ruled out. Autocorrelations can be adequately used for the purpose. It is a technique that cuts time curves into pieces. These pieces are, subsequently, compared with the original data-curve using linear regression analysis. Autocorrelation coefficients significantly larger and smaller than 0 must be observed in order to conclude periodicity. If not, spectral analysis is often helpful.

It displays a peak outcome at the frequency of the expected periodicity (months, years, weeks etc.). The current chapter shows that spectral analysis can be adequately used with very irregular patterns and inconclusive autocorrelation analysis, and is able to demonstrate unequivocal periodicities where visual methods like scatter-grams and traditional methods like autocorrelations are inconclusive.

A limitation of spectral analysis is the variance problem. The periodogram's variance does not decrease with increased sample sizes. However, smoothing using the spectral density function, is sample size dependent, and therefore, reduces the variance problem.

Note

More background, theoretical and mathematical information of spectral analysis and autocorrelations is given in Machine Learning in Medicine Part Three, Chap. 15, Spectral plots, pp. 151–160, Springer Heidelberg Germany 2013, and in Machine Learning in Medicine, Part One, Chap. 10, Seasonality assessments, pp. 113–126, Springer Heidelberg Germany, 2013, both from the same authors.

Chapter 10
Runs Test for Identifying Best Regression Models (21 Estimates of Quantity and Quality of Patient Care)

10.1 General Purpose

R-square values are often used to test the appropriateness of diagnostic models.

However, in practice, pretty large r-square values (squared correlation coefficients) may be observed even if data do not fit the model very well. This chapter assesses whether the runs test is a better alternative to the traditional r-square test for addressing the differences between the data and the best fit regression models.

10.2 Primary Scientific Question

A real data example was given comparing quantity of care with quality of care scores.

10.3 Example

Doctors were assessed for the relationship between their quantity and quality of care. The quantity of care was estimated with the numbers of daily interventions like endoscopies and small operations per doctor, the quality of care with quality of care scores. The data file is given below, and is also available in "runstest" on the internet at http://extras.springer.com.

© The Author(s) 2014
T.J. Cleophas and A.H. Zwinderman, *Machine Learning in Medicine—Cookbook Three*, SpringerBriefs in Statistics,
DOI 10.1007/978-3-319-12163-5_10

Quantity of care	Quality of care
19.00	2.00
20.00	3.00
23.00	4.00
24.00	5.00
26.00	6.00
27.00	7.00
28.00	8.00
29.00	9.00
29.00	10.00
29.00	11.00
28.00	12.00
27.00	13.00
27.00	14.00
26.00	15.00
25.00	16.00
24.00	17.00
23.00	18.00
22.00	19.00
22.00	20.00
21.00	21.00
21.00	22.00

Quantity of care numbers of daily interventions per doctor
Quality of care quality of care scores

The relationship seemed not to be linear, and curvilinear regression in SPSS was used to find the best fit curve to describe the data and eventually use them as prediction model. First, we will make a graph of the data.

Command:
Analyze…Graphs…Chart builder…click: Scatter/Dot…Click quality of care and drag to the Y-Axis…Click Intervention per doctor and drag to the X-Axis… OK.

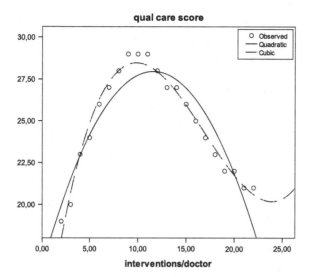

The above figure shows the scattergram of the data. A non-linear relationship is indeed suggested, and the curvilinear regression option in SPSS was helpful to find the best fit model.

Command:
Analyze...Regression...Curve Estimation...mark: Quadratic, Cubic...mark: Display ANOVA Table...OK.

The quadratic (best fit second order, parabolic, relationship) and cubic (best fit third order, hyperbolic, relationship) were the best options, with very good r-squares and p-values <0.0001 as shown in the table given by the software.

Model Summary and Parameter Estimates

Dependent Variable:qual care score

Equation	Model Summary					Parameter Estimates			
	R Square	F	df1	df2	Sig.	Constant	b1	b2	b3
Quadratic	0.866	58.321	2	18	0.000	16.259	2.017	−0.087	
Cubic	0.977	236.005	3	17	0.000	10.679	4.195	−0.301	0.006

The independent variable is interventions/doctor.

The runs test requires the residues from respectively the best fit quadratic and cubic models of the data (instead of − and + distances from the modeled curves (the residues) to be read from the above figure, the values 0 and 1 have to be added as separate variables in SPSS).

Quantity of care	Quality of care	Residues quadratic model	Residues cubic model
19.00	2.00	0.00	1.00
20.00	3.00	0.00	0.00
23.00	4.00	1.00	1.00
24.00	5.00	0.00	0.00
26.00	6.00	1.00	0.00
27.00	7.00	1.00	0.00
28.00	8.00	1.00	0.00
29.00	9.00	1.00	1.00
29.00	10.00	1.00	1.00
29.00	11.00	1.00	1.00
28.00	12.00	1.00	1.00
27.00	13.00	0.00	0.00
27.00	14.00	0.00	1.00
26.00	15.00	0.00	1.00
25.00	16.00	0.00	0.00
24.00	17.00	0.00	0.00
23.00	18.00	0.00	0.00
22.00	19.00	0.00	0.00
22.00	20.00	1.00	1.00
21.00	21.00	1.00	0.00
21.00	22.00	1.00	1.00

Command:
Analyze…Nonparametric tests…Runs Test…move the runsquadratic model residues variable to Test Variable List…click Options…click Descriptives… click Continue…click Cut Point…mark Median…click OK.

The output table shows that in the runs test the quadratic model differs from the actual data with $p = 0.02$. It means that the quadratic model is systematically different from the data.

Runs Test

	runsquadratic model
Test Value[a]	1.00
Cases < Test Value	10
Cases >= Test Value	11
Total Cases	21
Number of Runs	6
Z	−2.234
Asymp. Sig. (2-tailed)	0.026
Exact Sig. (2-tailed)	0.022
Point Probability	0.009

a. Median

When the similar procedure is followed for the best fit cubic model, the result is very insignificant with a p-value of 1.00. The cubic model was, thus, a much better predicting model for the data than the quadratic model.

Runs Test 2

	runscubicmodel
Test Value[a]	0.4762
Cases < Test Value	11
Cases >= Test Value	10
Total Cases	21
Number of Runs	11
Z	0.000
Asymp. Sig. (2-tailed)	1.000
Exact Sig. (2-tailed)	1.000
Point Probability	0.165

a. Mean

10.4 Conclusion

The runs test is appropriate both for testing whether fitted theoretical curves are systematically different or not from a given data set. The fit of regression models is traditionally assessed with r-square tests. However, the runs test is more appropriate for the purpose, because large r-square value do not exclude poor systematic data fit, and because the runs test assesses the entire pattern in the data, rather than mean distances between data and model.

Note
More background, theoretical and mathematical information of the runs test is given in Machine Learning in Medicine Part Three, Chap. 13, Runs test, pp. 127–135, Springer Heidelberg Germany 2013, from the same authors.

Chapter 11
Evolutionary Operations for Process Improvement (8 Operation Room Air Condition Settings)

11.1 General Purpose

Evolutionary operations (evops) try and find improved processes by exploring the effect of small changes in an experimental setting. It stems from evolutionary algorithms (see Machine Learning in Medicine Part Three, Chap. 2, Evolutionary Operations, pp. 11–18, Springer Heidelberg Germany, 2013, from the same authors), which uses rules based on biological evolution mechanisms where each next generation is slightly different and generally somewhat improved as compared to its ancestors. It is widely used not only in genetic research, but also in chemical and technical processes. So much so that the internet nowadays offers free evop calculators suitable not only for the optimization of the above processes, but also for the optimization of your pet's food, your car costs, and many other daily life standard issues. This chapter is to assess how evops can be helpful to optimize the air quality of operation rooms.

11.2 Specific Scientific Question

The air quality of operation rooms is important for infection prevention. Particularly, the factors (1) humidity (30–60 %), (2) filter capacity (70–90 %), and (3) air volume change (20–30 % per hour) are supposed to be important determinants. Can an evolutionary operation be used for process improvement.

© The Author(s) 2014
T.J. Cleophas and A.H. Zwinderman, *Machine Learning in Medicine—Cookbook Three*, SpringerBriefs in Statistics, DOI 10.1007/978-3-319-12163-5_11

11.3 Example

Eight operation room air condition settings were investigated, and the results are underneath.

Operation setting	Humidity (30 % = 1, 60 % = 4)	Filter capacity (70 % = 1, 90 % = 3)	Air volume change (20 % = 1, 30 % = 3)	Number of infections
1	1	1	1	99
2	2	1	1	90
3	1	2	1	75
4	2	2	1	73
5	1	1	2	99
6	2	1	2	99
7	1	2	2	61
8	2	2	2	52

We will use multiple linear regression in SPSS with the number of infections as outcome and the three factors as predictors to identify the significant predictors.

First, the data file available as "evops" in http://extras.springer.com is opened in SPSS.

Command:
Analyze…Regression…Linear…Dependent: enter "Var00004"…Independent (s): enter "Var00001-00003"…click OK.

The underneath table in the output shows that all of the determinants are statistically significant at $p < 0.10$. A higher humidity, filtering level, and air volume change better prevents infections.

Coefficients[a]

Model		Unstandardized Coefficients		Standardized Coefficients	t	Sig.
		B	Std. Error	Beta		
1	(Constant)	103.250	18.243		5.660	0.005
	hunidity1	−12.250	3.649	−0.408	−3.357	0.028
	filter capacity1	−21.250	3.649	−0.707	−5.824	0.004
	airvolume change1	15.750	3.649	0.524	4.317	0.012

a. Dependent Variable: infections1

In the next 8 operation settings higher determinant levels were assessed.

Operation setting	Humidity (30 % = 1, 60 % = 4)	Filter capacity (70 % = 1, 90 % = 3)	Air volume change (20 % = 1, 30 % = 3)	Number of infections
1	3	2	2	51
2	4	2	2	45
3	3	3	2	33
4	4	3	2	26
5	3	2	3	73
6	4	2	3	60
7	3	3	3	54
8	4	3	3	31

We will use again multiple linear regression in SPSS with the number of infections as outcome and the three factors as predictors to identify the significant predictors.

Command:

Analyze...Regression...Linear...Dependent: enter "Var00008"...Independent (s): enter "Var00005-00007"...click OK.

Coefficients[a]

Model		Unstandardized Coefficients		Standardized Coefficients	t	Sig.
		B	Std. Error	Beta		
1	(Constant)	145.500	15.512		9.380	0.001
	humidity2	−5.000	5.863	−0.145	−0.853	0.442
	filter capacity2	−31.500	5.863	−0.910	−5.373	0.006
	airvolume change2	−6.500	5.863	−0.188	−1.109	0.330

a. Dependent Variable: infections2

The underneath table in the output shows that only Var00006 (the filter capacity) is still statistically significant. Filter capacity 3 performs better than 2, while humidity levels and air volume changes were not significantly different. We could go one step further to find out how higher levels would perform, but for now we will conclude that humidity level 2–4, filter capacity level 3, and air flow change level 2–4 are efficacious level combinations. Higher levels of humidity and air flow change is not meaningful. An additional benefit of a higher level of filter capacity cannot be excluded, but requires additional testing.

11.4 Conclusion

Evolutionary operations can be used to improve the process of air quality maintenance in operation rooms. This methodology can similarly be applied for finding the best settings for numerous clinical, and laboratory settings. We have to add that interaction between the predictors was not taken into account in the current example. For a meaningful assessment of 2- and 3-factor interactions larger samples would be required, however. Moreover, we have clinical arguments that no important interactions are to be expected.

Note
More background, theoretical and mathematical information of evops is given in Machine Learning in Medicine, Part Three, Chap. 2, Evolutionary operations, pp. 11–18, Springer Heidelberg Germany, 2013, from the same authors.

Chapter 12
Bayesian Networks for Cause Effect Modeling (600 Patients Assessed for Longevity Factors)

12.1 General Purpose

Bayesian networks are probabilistic graphical models using nodes and arrows, respectively representing variables, and probabilistic dependencies between two variables. Computations in a Bayesian network are performed using weighted likelihood methodology and marginalization, meaning that irrelevant variables are integrated or summed out. Additional theoretical information is given in Machine Learning in Medicine Part Two, Chap. 16, Bayesian networks, pp. 163–170, Springer Heidelberg Germany, 2013, from the same authors. This chapter is to assess if Bayesian networks is able to determine direct and indirect predictors of binary outcomes like morbidity/mortality outcomes.

12.2 Primary Scientific Question

Longevity is multifactorial, and logistic regression is adequate to assess the chance of longevity in patients with various predictor scores like physical, psychological, and family scores. However, some factors may have both direct and indirect effects. Can a best fit Bayesian network demonstrate not only direct but also indirect effects of factors on the outcome?

© The Author(s) 2014
T.J. Cleophas and A.H. Zwinderman, *Machine Learning in Medicine—Cookbook Three*, SpringerBriefs in Statistics, DOI 10.1007/978-3-319-12163-5_12

12.3 Example

In 600 patients, 70 years of age, a score sampling of factors predicting longevity was performed. The outcome was death after 10 years of follow-up. The first 12 patients are underneath, the entire data file is in "longevity", and is available at http://extras.springer.com. We will first perform a logistic regression of these data using SPSS statistical software. Start by opening SPSS. Enter the above data file.

Variables					
1	2	3	4	5	6
Death	Econ	Psychol	Physic	Family	Educ
0	70	117	76	77	120
0	70	68	76	56	114
0	70	74	71	57	109
0	90	114	82	79	125
0	90	117	100	68	123
0	70	74	100	57	121
1	70	77	103	62	145
0	70	62	71	56	100
0	90	86	88	65	114
0	90	77	88	61	111
0	110	56	65	59	130
0	70	68	50	60	118

Death (0 no)
Econ economy score
Psychol psychological score
Physic physical score
Family familial risk score of longevity
Educ educational score

12.4 Binary Logistic Regression in SPSS

Command:
Analyze...Regression...Binary Logistic...Dependent: enter "death"...Covariates: enter "econ, psychol, physical, family, educ"...OK.

The underneath output table shows the results. With $p < 0.10$ as cut-off for statistical significance, all of the covariates, except economical score, were significant predictors of longevity (death), although both negative and positive b-values were observed.

Variables in the Equation

		B	S.E.	Wald	df	Sig.	Exp(B)
Step 1ᵃ	ecom	0.003	0.006	0.306	1	0.580	1.003
	psychol	−0.056	0.009	43.047	1	0.000	0.946
	physical	−0.019	0.007	8.589	1	0.003	0.981
	family	0.045	0.017	7.297	1	0.007	1.046
	educ	0.017	0.009	3.593	1	0.058	1.018
	Constant	−0.563	0.922	0.373	1	0.541	0.569

a. Variable(s) entered on step 1: ecom, psychol, physical, family, educ.

For these data we hypothesized that all of these scores would independently affect longevity. However, indirect effects were not taken into account, like the effect of psychological on physical scores, and the effect of family on educational scores etc. In order to assess both direct and indirect effects, a Bayesian network DAG (directed acyclic graph) was fitted to the data. The Konstanz Information Miner (Knime) was used for the analysis. In order to enter the SPSS data file in Knime, an excel version of the data file is required. For that purpose open the file in SPSS and follow the commands.

Command in SPSS:
click File...click Save as...in "Save as" type: enter Comma Delimited (*.csv)... click Save.

For convenience the excel file has been added to http://extras.springer.com, and is, just like the SPSS file, entitled "longevity".

12.5 Konstanz Information Miner (Knime)

In Google enter the term "knime". Click Download and follow instructions. After completing the pretty easy download procedure, open the knime workbench by clicking the knime welcome screen. The center of the screen displays the workflow editor like the canvas in SPSS Modeler. It is empty, and can be used to build a stream of nodes, called workflow in knime. The node repository is in the left lower angle of the screen, and the nodes can be dragged to the workflow editor simply by left-clicking. The nodes are computer tools for data analysis like visualization and statistical processes. Node description is in the right upper angle of the screen. Before the nodes can be used, they have to be connected with the file reader and with one another by arrows drawn again simply by left clicking the small triangles attached to the nodes. Right clicking on the file reader enables to configure from your computer a requested data file...click Browse...and download from the appropriate folder a csv type Excel file. You are almost set for analysis now, but in order to perform a Bayesian analysis Weka software 3.6 for windows (statistical software from the University of Waikato (New Zealand)) is required. Simply type the term Weka software, and find the site. The software can be freely downloaded from the internet, following a few simple instructions, and it can, subsequently, be readily opened in Knime. Once it has been opened, it is stored in your Knime node repository, and you will be able to routinely use it.

12.6 Knime Workflow

A knime workflow for the analysis of the above data example is built, and the final result is shown in the underneath figure, by dragging and connecting as explained above.

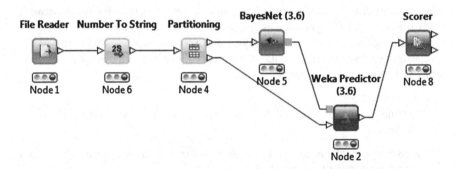

In the node repository click and type File Reader and drag to workflow editor in the node repository click again File reader...click the ESC button of your computer...in the node repository click again and type Number to String...the node is displayed...drag it to the workflow editor...perform the same kind of actions for all of the nodes as shown in the above figure...connect, by left clicking, all of the nodes with arrows as indicated above...click File Reader...click Browse...and type the requested data file ("longevity.csv")...click OK...the data file is given...right click all of the nodes and then right click Configurate and execute all of the nodes by right clicking the nodes and then the texts "Configurate" and "Execute"...the red lights will successively turn orange and then green...right click the Weka Predictor node...right click the Weka Node View...right click Graph.

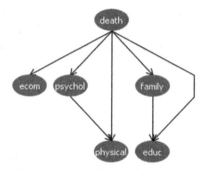

The above graph, a socalled directed acyclic graph (DAG) shows the Bayesian network obtained from the analysis. This best fitting DAG was, obviously, more complex than expected from the logistic model. Longevity was directly determined by all of the 5 predictors, but additional indirect effects were between physical and psychological scores, and between educational and family scores. In order to assess the validity of the Bayesian model, a confusion matrix and accuracy statistics were computed.

Right click the Scorer node…right click Confusion matrix.

12.6.1 Confusion Matrix

Table "spec_name" - Rows: 2	Spec - Columns: 2	Properties	Flow Variables
Row ID	**0**	**1**	
0	295	70	
1	91	44	

The observed and predicted values are summarized. Subsequently, right click Accuracy statistics.

12.6.2 Accuracy Statistics

Row ID	TruePo...	FalsePo...	TrueNe...	FalseN...	Recall	Precision	Sensitivity	Specifity
0	295	91	44	70	0.808	0.764	0.808	0.326
1	44	70	295	91	0.326	0.386	0.326	0.808
Overall	?	?	?	?	?	?	?	?

The sensitivity of the Bayesian model to predict longevity was pretty good, 80.8 %. However, the specificity was pretty bad. "No deaths" were rightly predicted in 80.8 % of the patients, "deaths", however, were rightly predicted in only 32.6 % of the patients.

12.7 Conclusion

Bayesian networks are probabilistic graphical models for assessing cause effect relationships. This chapter is to assess if Bayesian networks is able to determine direct and indirect predictors of binary outcomes like morbidity/mortality outcomes. As an example a longevity study is used. Longevity is multifactorial, and logistic regression is adequate to assess the chance of longevity in patients with various predictor scores like physical, psychological, and family scores. However, factors may have both direct and indirect effects. A best fit Bayesian network demonstrated not only direct but also indirect effects of the factors on the outcome.

Note
More background, theoretical and mathematical information of Bayesian networks is in Machine Learning in Medicine Part Two, Chap. 16, Bayesian networks, pp. 163–170, Springer Heidelberg Germany, 2013, from the same authors.

Chapter 13
Support Vector Machines for Imperfect Nonlinear Data (200 Patients with Sepsis)

13.1 General Purpose

The basic aim of support vector machines is to construct the best fit separation line (or with three dimensional data separation plane), separating cases and controls as good as possible. Discriminant analysis, classification trees, and neural networks (see Machine Learning in Medicine Part One, Chap. 17, Discriminant analysis for supervised data, pp. 215–224, Chap. 13, Artificial Intelligence, Chaps. 12 and 13, pp. 145–165, 2013, and Machine Learning in Medicine Part Three, Chap. 14, Decision Trees, pp. 137–150, 2013, Springer Heidelberg Germany, by the same authors as the current chapter) are alternative methods for the purpose, but support vector machines are generally more stable and sensitive, although heuristic studies to indicate when they perform better are missing. Support vector machines are also often used in automatic modeling that computes the ensembled results of several best fit models (see Machine Learning in Medicine Cookbook Two, Chaps. 18 and 19, Automatic modeling of drug efficacy prediction, and Automatic modeling for clinical event prediction, pp. 99–111, 2014, Springer Heidelberg Germany, from the same authors). This chapter uses the Konstanz Information Miner, a free data mining software package developed at the University of Konstanz, and also used in the Chaps. 1 and 2.

13.2 Primary Scientific Question

Is support vector machines adequate to classify cases and controls in a cohort of admitted because of sepsis?

© The Author(s) 2014
T.J. Cleophas and A.H. Zwinderman, *Machine Learning in Medicine—Cookbook Three*, SpringerBriefs in Statistics, DOI 10.1007/978-3-319-12163-5_13

13.3 Example

Two hundred patients were admitted because of sepsis. The laboratory values and
the outcome death or alive were registered. We wish to use support vector machines
to predict from the laboratory values the outcome, death or alive, including information on the error rate. The data of the first 12 patients are underneath. The entire
data file is in http://extras.springer.com. Konstanz Information Miner (KNIME)
does not use SPSS files, and, so, the file has to be transformed into a csv excel file
(click Save As...in "Save as" type: replace SPSS Statistics(*sav) with SPSS Sta-
tistics(*csv). For convenience the csv file is in http://extras.springer.com and is
entitled "svm".

Death	Ggt	asat	alat	bili	ureum	creat	c-clear	esr	crp	leucos
1 = yes										
Var1	Var2	Var3	Var4	Var5	Var6	Var7	Var8	Var9	Var10	Var11
0	20	23	34	2	3.4	89	−111	2	2	5
0	14	21	33	3	2	67	−112	7	3	6
0	30	35	32	4	5.6	58	−116	8	4	4
0	35	34	40	4	6	76	−110	6	5	7
0	23	33	22	4	6.1	95	−120	9	6	6
0	26	31	24	3	5.4	78	−132	8	4	8
0	15	29	26	2	5.3	47	−120	12	5	5
0	13	26	24	1	6.3	65	−132	13	6	6
0	26	27	27	4	6	97	−112	14	6	7
0	34	25	13	3	4	67	−125	15	7	6
0	32	26	24	3	3.6	58	−110	13	8	6
0	21	13	15	3	3.6	69	−102	12	2	4

Var1 death 1 yes
Var2 gammagt (Var variable) (U/l)
Var3 asat (U/l)
Var4 alat (U/l)
Var5 bili (μmol/l)
Var6 ureum (mmol/l)
Var7 creatinine (μmol/l)
Var8 creatinine clearance (ml/min)
Var9 esr (erythrocyte sedimentation rate) (mm)
Var10 c-reactive protein (mg/l)
Var11 leucos ($\times 10^9$ /l)

13.4 Knime Data Miner

In Google enter the term "knime". Click Download and follow instructions. After
completing the pretty easy download procedure, open the knime workbench by
clicking the knime welcome screen. The center of the screen displays the workflow
editor like the canvas in SPSS Modeler. It is empty, and can be used to build a
stream of nodes, called workflow in knime. The node repository is in the left lower

angle of the screen, and the nodes can be dragged to the workflow editor simply by left-clicking. The nodes are computer tools for data analysis like visualization and statistical processes. Node description is in the right upper angle of the screen. Before the nodes can be used they have to be connected with the file reader and with one another by arrows drawn again simply by left clicking the small triangles attached to the nodes. Right clicking on the file reader enables to configure from your computer a requested data file.

13.5 Knime Workflow

A knime workflow for the analysis of the above data example will be built, and the final result is shown in the underneath figure.

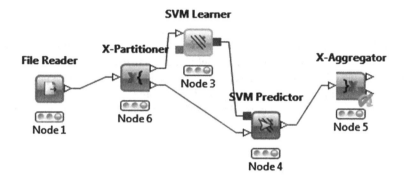

13.6 File Reader Node

In the node repository find the node File Reader. Drag the node to the workflow editor by left clicking...click Browse...and download from http://extras.springer.com the csv type Excel file entitled "svm". You are set for analysis now. By left clicking the node the file is displayed. The File Reader has chosen Var0006 (ureum) as S variable (dependent). However, we wish to replace it with Var0001 (death yes = 1)...click the column header of Var0006...mark "Don't include column in output"...click OK...in the column header of Var0001 leave unmarked "Don't include column in output" click OK.

The outcome variable is now rightly the Var0001 and is indicated with S, the Var0006 has obtained the term "SKIP" between brackets.

13.7 The Nodes X-Partitioner, SVM Learner, SVM Predictor, X-Aggregator

Find the above nodes in the node repository and drag them to the workflow editor and connect them with one another according to the above figure. Configurate and execute all them by right clicking the nodes and the texts "Configurate" and "Execute". The red lights under the nodes get, subsequently, yellow and, then, green. The miner has accomplished its task.

13.8 Error Rates

Right click the X-Aggregator node once more, and then right click Error rates. The underneath table is shown. The svm model is used to make predictions about death or not from the other variables of your file. Nine random samples of 25 patients are shown. The error rates are pretty small, and vary from 0 to 12.5 %. We should add that other measures of uncertainty like sensitivity or specificity are not provided by knime.

Row ID	D Error in %	｜ Size of ...	｜ Error C...
fold 0	4	25	1
fold 1	4	25	1
fold 2	4.167	24	1
fold 3	12	25	3
fold 4	4.167	24	1
fold 5	8	25	2
fold 6	12	25	3
fold 7	0	24	0
fold 8	8	25	2
fold 9	12.5	24	3

Error rates - 0:5 - X-Aggregator

File

Table "default" - Rows: 10 | Spec - Columns: 3 | Properties | Flow Variables

13.9 Prediction Table

Right click the X-Aggregator node once more, and then right click Prediction Table. The underneath table is shown. The svm model is used to make predictions about death or not from the other variables of your file.

The left column gives the outcome values (death yes = 1), the right one gives the predicted values. It can be observed that the two results very well match one another.

Prediction table - 0:5 - X-Aggregator

File

Table "default" - Rows: 246 | Spec - Columns: 11 | Properties | Flow Variables

Row ID	S i>cVAR...	VAR00...	VAR00...	VAR00...	VAR00...	VAR00...	VAR00...	VAR00...	VAR00...	VAR00...	S Predicti...
Row4	0	23	33	22	4	95	-120	9	6	6	0
Row6	0	15	29	26	2	47	-120	12	5	5	0
Row9	0	34	25	13	3	67	-125	15	7	6	0
Row14	0	19	16	9	4	80	-113	8	4	7	0
Row18	0	24	24	27	4	84	-120	15	6	6	0
Row36	0	19	236	15	2	78	-113	7	6	6	0
Row42	0	27	17	27	4	98	-101	14	4	3	0
Row47	0	15	17	15	2	89	-112	13	9	6	0
Row62	0	16	14	19	4	67	-102	14	7	2	0
Row64	0	14	14	27	2	76	-109	18	5	5	0
Row66	0	16	27	29	3	77	-102	14	4	6	0
Row67	0	24	25	24	2	69	-110	16	5	7	0
Row68	0	21	29	25	4	78	-112	15	7	4	0
Row73	0	21	15	13	2	92	-120	17	7	4	0
Row114	1	900	759	856	287	532	-8	109	103	23	1
Row144	1	376	459	389		267	-29	97	33	20	1
Row151	1	169	154	267	75	244	-50	42	21	15	1
Row155	1	175	250	276	95	231	-41	36	28	15	1
Row170	1	276	230	156	79	235	-54	34	23	15	1
Row181	1	75	84	145	39	137	-66	28	18	14	1

13.10 Conclusion

The basic aim of support vector machines is to construct the best fit separation line (or with three dimensional data separation plane), separating cases and controls as good as possible. This chapter uses the Konstanz Information Miner, a free data mining software package developed at the University of Konstanz, and also used in the Chaps. 1 and 2. The example shows that support vector machines is adequate to predict the presence of a disease or not in a cohort of patients at risk of a disease.

Note

More background, theoretical and mathematical information of support vector machines is given in Machine in Medicine Part Two, Chap. 14, Support vector machines, pp. 155–162, 2–13, Springer Heidelberg Germany, from the same authors.

Chapter 14
Multiple Response Sets for Visualizing Clinical Data Trends (811 Patient Visits to General Practitioners)

14.1 General Purpose

Multiple response methodology answers multiple qualitative questions about a single group of patients, and uses for the purpose summary tables. The method visualizes trends and similarities in the data, but no statistical test is given.

14.2 Specific Scientific Question

Can multiple response sets better than traditional frequency tables demonstrate results that could be selected for formal trend tests.

14.3 Example

An 811 person health questionnaire addressed the reasons for visiting general practitioners (gps) in 1 month. Nine qualitative questions addressed various aspects of health as primary reasons for visits. SPSS statistical software was used to analyze the data.

© The Author(s) 2014
T.J. Cleophas and A.H. Zwinderman, *Machine Learning
in Medicine—Cookbook Three*, SpringerBriefs in Statistics,
DOI 10.1007/978-3-319-12163-5_14

Ill	Alcohol	Weight	Tired	Cold	Family	Mental	Physical	Social	No
0	0	1	1	0	0	0	0	1	0
1	1	1	1	1	1	1	1	1	0
0	0	0	0	0	0	0	0	0	1
1	0	0	1	0	0	0	0	0	0
1	0	0	0	1	1	1	1	0	0
0	0	0	0	0	1	1	1	0	0
0	0	0	0	0	0	0	0	0	1
1	1	0	1	1	1	1	1	1	0
0	0	0	0	0	0	1	0	0	0
1	1	0	1	0	1	1	1	1	0
0	0	0	0	0	0	0	0	0	1
0	0	0	0	0	1	1	1	0	0
1	1	0	1	1	1	0	1	1	0
1	0	0	0	1	0	1	0	0	0
1	0	0	1	0	0	0	1	1	0

Ill ill feeling
Alcohol alcohol abuse
Weight weight problems
Tired tiredness
Cold common cold
Family family problem
Mental mental problem
Physical physical problem
Social social problem
No no answer

The first 15 patient data are given. The entire data file is entitled "multipleresponse", and can be downloaded from www.springer.com. SPSS statistical software is used for analysis. We will start by the descriptive statistics.

Command:
Descriptive Statistics...Frequencies...Variables: enter the variables between "illfeeling" to "no answer"...click Statistics...click Sum...click Continue... click OK.

The output is in the underneath 10 tables. It is pretty hard to observe trends across the tables. Also redundant information as given is not helpful for overall conclusion about the relationships between the different questions.

ill feeling

		Frequency	Percent	Valid Percent	Cumulative Percent
Valid	No	420	43.3	51.8	51.8
	Yes	391	40.3	48.2	100.0
	Total	811	83.6	100.0	
Missing	System	159	16.4		
Total		970	100.0		

alcohol

		Frequency	Percent	Valid Percent	Cumulative Percent
Valid	No	569	58.7	70.2	70.2
	Yes	242	24.9	29.8	100.0
	Total	811	83.6	100.0	
Missing	System	159	16.4		
Total		970	100.0		

weight problem

		Frequency	Percent	Valid Percent	Cumulative Percent
Valid	No	597	61.5	73.6	73.6
	Yes	214	22.1	26.4	100.0
	Total	811	83.6	100.0	
Missing	System	159	16.4		
Total		970	100.0		

tiredness

		Frequency	Percent	Valid Percent	Cumulative Percent
Valid	No	511	52.7	63.0	63.0
	Yes	300	30.9	37.0	100.0
	Total	811	83.6	100.0	
Missing	System	159	16.4		
Total		970	100.0		

cold

		Frequency	Percent	Valid Percent	Cumulative Percent
Valid	No	422	43.5	52.0	52.0
	Yes	389	40.1	48.0	100.0
	Total	811	83.6	100.0	
Missing	System	159	16.4		
Total		970	100.0		

family problem

		Frequency	Percent	Valid Percent	Cumulative Percent
Valid	No	416	42.9	51.3	51.3
	Yes	395	40.7	48.7	100.0
	Total	811	83.6	100.0	
Missing	System	159	16.4		
Total		970	100.0		

mental problem

		Frequency	Percent	Valid Percent	Cumulative Percent
Valid	No	410	42.3	50.6	50.6
	Yes	401	41.3	49.4	100.0
	Total	811	83.6	100.0	
Missing	System	159	16.4		
Total		970	100.0		

physical problem

		Frequency	Percent	Valid Percent	Cumulative Percent
Valid	No	402	41.4	49.6	49.6
	Yes	409	42.2	50.4	100.0
	Total	811	83.6	100.0	
Missing	System	159	16.4		
Total		970	100.0		

social problem

		Frequency	Percent	Valid Percent	Cumulative Percent
Valid	No	518	53.4	63.9	63.9
	Yes	293	30.2	36.1	100.0
	Total	811	83.6	100.0	
Missing	System	159	16.4		
Total		970	100.0		

no answer

		Frequency	Percent	Valid Percent	Cumulative Percent
Valid	0.00	722	74.4	89.0	89.0
	1.00	89	9.2	11.0	100.0
	Total	811	83.6	100.0	
Missing	System	159	16.4		
Total		970	100.0		

In order to find out more about trends in the data a multiple response analysis will be performed next.

Command:
Analyze...Multiple Response...Define Variable Sets...move "ill feeling, alcohol, tiredness, cold, family problem, mental problem, physical problem, social problem" from Set Definition to Variables in Set...Counted Values enter 1... Name enter "health"...Label enter "health"...Multiple Response Set: click Add...click Close...click Analyze...Multiple Response...click Frequencies ... move $health from Multiple Response Sets to Table(s)...click OK.

The underneath Case Summary table show that of all visitants 25.6 % did not answer any question, here called the missing cases.

Case Summary

	Cases					
	Valid		Missing		Total	
	N	Percent	N	Percent	N	Percent
$health^a	722	74.4%	248	25.6%	970	100.0%

a. Dichotomy group tabulated at value 1.

$health Frequencies

		Responses		Percent of Cases
		N	Percent	
health^a	ill feeling	391	12.9%	54.2%
	alcohol	242	8.0%	33.5%
	weight problem	214	7.1%	29.6%
	tiredness	300	9.9%	41.6%
	cold	389	12.8%	53.9%
	family problem	395	13.0%	54.7%
	mental problem	401	13.2%	55.5%
	physical problem	409	13.5%	56.6%
	social problem	293	9.7%	40.6%
Total		3034	100.0%	420.2%

a. Dichotomy group tabulated at value 1.

The letter N gives the numbers of yes-answers per question, "Percent of Cases" gives the yes-answers per question in those who answered at least once (missing data not taken into account), and Percent gives the percentages of these yes-answers per question.

The above output shows the number of patients who answered yes to at least one question. Of all visitants 25.6 % did not answer any question, here called the missing cases. In the second table the letter N gives the numbers of yes-answers per question, "Percent of Cases" gives the yes-answers per question in those who answered at least once (missing data not taken into account), and "Percent" gives the percentages of these yes-answers per question. The gp consultation burden of mental and physical problems was about twice the size of that of alcohol and weight problems. Tiredness and social problems were in-between. In order to assess these data against all visitants, the missing cases have to be analyzed first.

Command:
Transform...Compute Variable...Target Variable: type "none"...Numeric Expression: enter "1-max(illfeeling, ..., social problem)" ...click Type and Label...LabelL enter "no answer"...click Continue...click OK...Analyze... Multiple Response...Define Variable sets...click Define Multiple Response

Sets…click $health…move "no answer" to Variables in Set…click Change… click Close.

The data file now contains the novel "no answer" variable and a novel multiple response variable including the missing cases but the latter is not shown. It is now also possible to produce crosstabs with the different questions as rows and other variables like personal characteristics as columns. In this way the interaction with the personal characteristics can be assessed.

Command:
Analyze…Multiple Response…Multiple Response Crosstabs…Rows: enter $health…Columns: enter ed (= level of education)…click Define Range… Minimum: enter 1…Maximum: enter 5…Continue…Click Options…Cell Percentages: click Columns…click Continue…click OK.

$health*ed Crosstabulation

			Level of education					
			no highschool	highschool	college	university	completed university	Total
health[a]	ill feeling	Count	45	101	87	115	43	391
		% within ed	27.6%	43.3%	50.9%	60.2%	81.1%	
	alcohol	Count	18	55	52	83	34	242
		% within ed	11.0%	23.6%	30.4%	43.5%	64.2%	
	weight problem	Count	13	51	43	82	25	214
		% within ed	8.0%	21.9%	25.1%	42.9%	47.2%	
	tiredness	Count	10	55	71	122	42	300
		% within ed	6.1%	23.6%	41.5%	63.9%	79.2%	
	cold	Count	71	116	85	96	21	389
		% within ed	43.6%	49.8%	49.7%	50.3%	39.6%	
	family problem	Count	75	118	84	93	25	395
		% within ed	46.0%	50.6%	49.1%	48.7%	47.2%	
	mental problem	Count	78	112	91	94	26	401
		% within ed	47.9%	48.1%	53.2%	49.2%	49.1%	
	physical problem	Count	78	123	87	95	26	409
		% within ed	47.9%	52.8%	50.9%	49.7%	49.1%	
	social problem	Count	11	67	68	111	36	293
		% within ed	6.7%	28.8%	39.8%	58.1%	67.9%	
	no answer	Count	39	29	13	6	2	89
		% within ed	23.9%	12.4%	7.6%	3.1%	3.8%	
Total		Count	163	233	171	191	53	811

Percentages and totals are based on respondents.

a. Dichotomy group tabulated at value 1.

The output table gives the results. Various trends are observed. E.g., there is a decreasing trend of patients not answering any question with increased levels of education. Also there is an increasing trend of ill feeling, alcohol problems, weight problems, tiredness and social problems with increased levels of education. If we wish to test whether the increasing trend of tiredness with increased level of education is statistically significant, a formal trend test can be performed.

Command:
Analyze...Descriptive Statistics...Crosstabs...Rows: enter tiredness...Columns: enter level of education...click Statistics...mark Chi-square...click Continue... click OK.

Underneath a formal trend test is given. It tests whether an increasing trend of tiredness is associated with increased levels of education.

Chi-Square Tests

	Value	df	Asymp. Sig. (2-sided)
Pearson Chi-Square	185.824[a]	4	0.000
Likelihood Ratio	202.764	4	0.000
Linear-by-Linear Association	184.979	1	0.000
N of Valid Cases	811		

a. 0 cells (0.0%) have expected count less than 5. The minimum expected count is 19.61.

In the output chi-square tests are given. The linear-by-linear association data show a chi-square value of 184.979 and 1 degree of freedom. This means that a statistically very significant linear trend with $p < 0.0001$ is in these data.

Also interactions and trends of any other health problems with all of the other variables including gender, age, marriage, income, period of constant address or employment can be similarly analyzed.

14.4 Conclusion

The answers to a set of multiple questions about a single underlying disease/ condition can be assessed as multiple dimensions of a complex variable. Multiple response methodology is adequate for the purpose. The most important advantage of the multiple response methodology versus traditional frequency table analysis is that it is possible to observe relevant trends and similarities directly from data tables. A disadvantage is that only summaries but no statistical tests are given, but observed trends can, of course, be, additionally, tested statistically with formal trend tests.

Note
More background, theoretical and mathematical information of multiple response sets are in Machine Learning in Medicine Part Three, Chap. 11, pp. 105–115, Multiple response sets, Springer Heidelberg Germany, 2014, from the same authors.

Chapter 15
Protein and DNA Sequence Mining

15.1 General Purpose

Sequence similaritysearching is a method that can be applied by almost anybody for finding similarities between his/her query sequences of amino acids and DNA and the sequences known to be associated with different clinical effects. The latter have been included in database systems like the Basic Local Alignment Search Tool (BLAST) database system from the US National Center of Biotechnology Information (NCBI), and the MOTIF data base system, a joint website from different European and American institutions, and they are available through the internet for the benefit of individual researchers trying and finding a match for novel sequences from their own research. This chapter is to demonstrate that sequence similarity searching is a method that can be applied by almost anybody for finding similarities between his/her sequences and the sequences known to be associated with different clinical effects.

© The Author(s) 2014
T.J. Cleophas and A.H. Zwinderman, *Machine Learning in Medicine—Cookbook Three*, SpringerBriefs in Statistics, DOI 10.1007/978-3-319-12163-5_15

15.2 Specific Scientific Question

Abbreviations for amino acids

Amino acid	Three-letter abbreviation	One-letter symbol
Alanine	Ala	A
Arginine	Arg	R
Asparagine	Asn	N
Aspartic acid	Asp	D
Asparagine or aspartic acid	Asx	B
Cysteine	Cys	C
Glutamine	Gln	Q
Glutamic acid	Glu	E
Glutamine or glutamic acid	Glx	Z
Glycine	Gly	G
Histidine	His	H
Isoleucine	Ile	I
Leucine	Leu	L
Lysine	Lys	K
Methionine	Met	M
Phenylalanine	Phe	F
Proline	Pro	P
Serine	Ser	S
Threonine	Thr	T
Tryptophan	Trp	W
Tyrosine	Tyr	Y
Valine	Val	V

In this chapter amino acid sequences are analyzed, but nucleic acids sequences can similarly be assessed. The above table gives the one letter abbreviations of amino acids. The specific scientific question is: can sequence similarity search be applied for finding similarities between the sequences found in your own research and the sequences known to be associated with different clinical effects.

15.3 Data Base Systems on the Internet

The BLAST (http://blast.ncbi.nlm.nih.gov/Blast.cgi) program reports several terms:

1. Max score = best bit score between query sequence and database sequence (the bit score = the standardized score, i.e. the score that is independent of any unit).
2. Total score = best bit score if some amino acid pairs in the data have been used more often than just once.

3. Query coverage = percentage of amino acids used in the analysis.
4. E-value = expected number of large similarity alignment scores.

If the E-value is very small for the score observed, then a chance finding can be rejected. The sequences are then really related. An E-value = p-value adjusted for multiple testing = the chance that the association found is a chance finding. It indicates that the match between a novel and already known sequence is closer than could happen by chance, and that the novel and known sequence are thus homologous (philogenetically from the same ancestor, whatever that means).

15.4 Example 1

We isolated the following amino acid sequence: serine, isoleucine, lysine, leucine, tryptophan, proline, proline. The one letter abbreviation code for this sequence is SIKLWPP. The BLAST Search site is explored, while giving the following commands.

Open BLAST Search site at appropriate address (Reference 1).
Choose Protein BLAST
Click Enter Sequences and enter the amino acid sequence SIKLWPP
Click BLAST

The output tables use the term blast hit which means here a database sequence selected by the provider's software to be largely similar to the unknown sequence, and the term query, which means here an unknown sequence that the investigator has entered for sequence testing against known sequences from the database. The output tables report

1. No putative conserved domains have been detected.
2. In the Distribution of 100 Blast Hits on the Query sequence all of the Blast Hits have a very low alignment score (<40).
3. In spite of the low scores their precise alignment values are given next, e.g. the best one has

a max score of 21.8,
total score of 21.8,
query coverage of 100 %, and
adjusted p-value of 1,956 (not significant).

As a contrast search the MOTIF Search site is explored. We command.

Open MOTIF Search site at appropriate address (MOTIF Search. http://www.genome.jp/tools/motif).
Choose: Searching Protein Sequence Motifs
Click: Enter your query sequence and enter the amino acid sequence SIKLWPP
Select motif libraries: click various databases given
Then click Search.

The output table reports: 1 motif found in PROSITE database (found motif PKC_PHOSPHO_SITE; description: protein kinase C phosphorylation site). Obviously, it is worthwhile to search other databases if one does not provide any hits.

15.5 Example 2

We wish to examine a 12 amino acid sequence that we isolated at our laboratory, use again BLAST. We command.

Open BLAST Search site at appropriate address (Reference 1).
Choose Protein BLAST
Click Enter Sequences and enter the amino acid sequence ILVFMCWLVFQC
Click BLAST

The output tables report

1. No putative conserved domains have been detected.
2. In the Distribution of 100 Blast Hits on the Query sequence all of the Blast Hits have a very low alignment score (<40).
3. In spite of the low scores their precise alignment values are given next. Three of them have a significant alignment score at $p < 0.05$ with

> max scores of 31.2,
> total scores 31.2,
> query cover of around 60 %, and
> E-values (adjusted p-values) of 4.1, 4.1, and 4.5.

Parts of the novel sequence have been aligned to known sequences of proteins from a Streptococcus and a Nocardia bacteria and from Caenorhabditis, a small soil-dwelling nematode. These findings may not seem clinically very relevant, and may be due to type I errors, with low levels of statistical significance, or material contamination.

15.6 Example 3

A somewhat larger amino acid sequence (25 letters) is examined using BLAST. We command.

Open BLAST Search site at appropriate address (Reference 1).
Choose Protein BLAST
Click Enter Sequences and enter the amino acid sequence
SIKLWPPSQTTRLLLVERMANNLST
Click BLAST

The output tables report the following.

1. Putative domains have been detected. Specific hits regard the WPP superfamily. The WPP domain is a 90 amino acid protein that serves as a transporter protein for other protein in the plant cell from the cell plasma to the nucleus.
2. In the Distribution of 100 Blast Hits on the Query sequence all of the Blast Hits have a very high alignment score (80–200 for the first 5 hits, over 50 for the remainder, all of them statistically very significant).
3. Precise alignment values are given next. The first 5 hits have the highest scores: with

   > max scores of 83.8,
   > total scores of 83.8,
   > Cover queries of 100 %,
   > p-values of $4e^{-17}$, which is much smaller than 0.05 (5 %).

   All of them relate to the WPP superfamily sequence.
   The next 95 hits produced Max scores and Total scores from 68.9 to 62.1, query coverages from 100 to 96 % and adjusted p-values from $5e^{-12}$ to $1e^{-9}$, which is again much smaller than 0.05 (5 %).
4. We can subsequently browse through the 95 hits to see if anything of interest for our purposes can be found. All of the alignments as found regarded plant proteins like those of grasses, maize, nightshade and other plants, no alignments with human or veterinary proteins were established.

15.7   Example 4

A 27 amino acid sequence from a laboratory culture of pseudomonas is examined using BLAST. We command.

> Open BLAST Search site at appropriate address (Reference 1).
> Choose Protein BLAST
> Click Enter Sequences and enter the amino acid sequence MTDLNIPHT HAHLVDAFQALGIRAQAL
> Click BLAST

The output tables report

1. No putative domains have been detected.
2. The 100 blast hit table shows, however, a very high alignment score for gentamicin acetyl transferase enzyme, recently recognized as being responsible for resistance of Pseudomonas to gentamicin. The ailments values were

   > max score
   > total score of 85.5,
   > query coverage of 100 %,
   > adjusted p-value of $1e^{-17}$, and so statistically very significant.

3. In the Distribution of the 99 remaining Blast Hits only 5 other significant
   alignment were detected with

   max score and total scores from 38.5 to 32.9,
   query coverages 55–92 %,
   adjusted *p*-values between 0.08 and 4.5 (all of them 5 %).

   The significant alignments regarded bacterial proteins including the gram negative bacteria, rhizobium, xanthomonas, and morganella, and a mite protein. This
may not clinically be very relevant, but our novel sequence was derived from a
pseudomonas culture, and we know now that this particular culture contains
pathogens very resistant to gentamicin.

15.8 Conclusion

Sequence similarity searching is a method that can be applied by almost anybody
for finding similarities between his/her query sequences and the sequences known
to be associated with different clinical effects.

   With sequence similarity searching the use of *p*-values to distinguish between
high and low similarity is relevant. Unlike the BLAST interactive website, the
MOTIF interactive website does not give them, which hampers inferences from the
alignments to be made.

Note

More background, theoretical and mathematical information of protein and DNA
sequence mining is given in Machine Learning in Medicine Part Two, Chap. 17,
pp. 171–185, Protein and DNA sequence mining, Springer Heidelberg Germany
2013, from the same authors.

Chapter 16
Iteration Methods for Crossvalidations (150 Patients with Pneumonia)

16.1 General Purpose

In Chap. 2 of this volume validation of a decision tree model is performed splitting a data file into a training and a testing sample. This method performed pretty well with a sensitivity of 90–100 % and an overall accuracy of 94 %. However, measures of error of predictive models like the above one are based on residual methods, assuming a priori defined data distributions, particularly normal distributions. Machine learning data file may not meet such assumptions, and distribution free methods of validation, like crossvalidations may be more safe.

16.2 Primary Scientific Question

How does crossvalidation of the data from Chap. 3 perform as compared to the residual method used in the scorer node of the Konstanz Information Miner (Knime)?

16.3 Example

The data file from Chap. 2 is used once more. Four inflammatory markers [C-reactive protein (CRP), erythrocyte sedimentation rate (ESR), leucocyte count (leucos), and fibrinogen] were measured in 150 patients. Based on X-ray chest

© The Author(s) 2014
T.J. Cleophas and A.H. Zwinderman, *Machine Learning in Medicine—Cookbook Three*, SpringerBriefs in Statistics, DOI 10.1007/978-3-319-12163-5_16

clinical severity was classified as A (mild infection), B (medium severity), C (severe infection). A major scientific question was to assess what markers were the best predictors of the severity of infection.

CRP	Leucos'	Fibrinogen	ESR	X-ray severity
120.00	5.00	11.00	60.00	A
100.00	5.00	11.00	56.00	A
94.00	4.00	11.00	60.00	A
92.00	5.00	11.00	58.00	A
100.00	5.00	11.00	52.00	A
108.00	6.00	17.00	48.00	A
92.00	5.00	14.00	48.00	A
100.00	5.00	11.00	54.00	A
88.00	5.00	11.00	54.00	A
98.00	5.00	8.00	60.00	A
108.00	5.00	11.00	68.00	A
96.00	5.00	11.00	62.00	A
96.00	5.00	8.00	46.00	A
86.00	4.00	8.00	60.00	A
116.00	4.00	11.00	50.00	A
114.00	5.00	17.00	52.00	A

CRP C-reactive protein (mg/l)
Leucos leucocyte count ($*10^9$/l)
Fibrinogen fibrinogen level (mg/l)
ESR erythrocyte sedimentation rate (mm)
X-ray severity X-chest severity pneumonia score (A − C = mild to severe)

The first 16 patients are in the above table, the entire data file is in "decisiontree" and can be obtained from "http://extras.springer.com" on the internet.

16.4 Downloading the Knime Data Miner

In Google enter the term "knime". Click Download and follow instructions. After completing the pretty easy download procedure, open the knime workbench by clicking the knime welcome screen. The center of the screen displays the workflow editor like the canvas in SPSS Modeler. It is empty, and can be used to build a stream of nodes, called workflow in knime. The node repository is in the left lower angle of the screen, and the nodes can be dragged to the workflow editor simply by left-clicking. Start by dragging the file reader node to the workflow. The nodes are computer tools for data analysis like visualization and statistical processes. Node description is in the right upper angle of the screen. Before the nodes can be used, they have to be connected with the file reader node and with one another by arrows drawn again simply by left clicking the small triangles attached to the nodes. Right clicking on the file reader node enables to configure from your computer a requested data file...click Browse...and download from the appropriate folder a csv type Excel file. You are set for analysis now.

Note: the above data file cannot be read by the file reader node as it is an SPSS file, and must first be saved as an csv type Excel file. For that purpose command in SPSS: click File...click Save as...in "Save as type: enter Comma Delimited (*.csv)"...click Save. For your convenience it is available in www.springer.com, and is also entitled "decisiontree".

16.5 Knime Workflow

A knime workflow for the analysis of the above data example is built, and the final result is shown in the underneath figure.

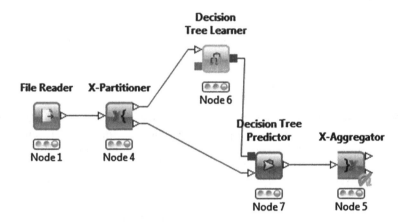

In the node repository click X-Partitioner, Decision Tree Learner, Decision Tree Predictor and X-Aggregator and drag them to the workflow editor. If you have difficulty finding the nodes (the repository contains hundreds of nodes), you may type their names in the small window at the top of the node repository box, and its icon and name will immediately appear. Connect, by left clicking, all of the nodes with arrows as indicated above...Configurate and execute all of the nodes by right clicking the nodes and then the texts "Configurate" and "Execute"...the red lights will successively turn orange and then green...right click the Decision Tree Predictor again...right click the text "View: Decision Tree View". The decision tree comes up, and it is, obviously, identical to the one of Chap. 2.

16.6 Crossvalidation

If you, subsequently, right click the Decision Tree Predictor, and then click Classified Data, a table turns up of 15 randomly selected subjects from your test sample. The predicted values are identical to the measured ones. And, so, for this selection the Decision Tree Predictor node performed well.

Row ID	i»¿CRP	leucos	fibrinogen	ESR	S xrayse...	S Predicti...
Row5	108	6	17	48	A	A
Row20	108	6	11	60	A	A
Row28	104	4	11	58	A	A
Row39	102	5	11	56	A	A
Row94	112	14	44	76	B	B
Row103	126	19	59	68	C	C
Row111	128	18	62	70	C	C
Row112	136	18	68	72	C	C
Row113	114	17	65	60	C	C
Row120	138	19	74	99	C	C
Row126	124	16	59	84	C	C
Row137	128	18	59	44	C	C
Row138	120	16	59	98	C	C
Row144	134	19	80	100	C	C
Row145	134	17	74	64	C	C

Next, right click the X-Aggregator node, and then click Prediction table. The results of 10 iterative random samples of 15 subjects from your test sample are simultaneously displayed. Obviously, virtually all of the predictions were in agreement with the measured values. Subsequently, right click the node again, and then click Error rates.

Error rates - 0:5 - X-Aggregator

File

Table "default" - Rows: 10   Spec - Columns: 3   Properties   Flow Variables

Row ID	D Error in %	I Size of ...	I Error C...
fold 0	6.667	15	1
fold 1	6.667	15	1
fold 2	6.667	15	1
fold 3	20	15	3
fold 4	0	15	0
fold 5	0	15	0
fold 6	6.667	15	1
fold 7	6.667	15	1
fold 8	0	15	0
fold 9	0	15	0

The above table comes up. It shows the error rates of the above 10 iterative random samples. The result is pretty good. Virtually, all of them have 0 or 1 erroneous value.

The crossvalidation can also be performed with a novel validation set. For that purpose you need a novel file reader node, and the novel validation set has to be configured and executed. Furthermore, you need to copy and paste the above Aggregator node, and you need to connect the output port of the above Decision Tree Predictor node to the input port of Aggregator node.

16.7 Conclusion

In Chap. 2 of this volume validation of a decision tree model was performed splitting a data file into a training and testing sample. This method performed pretty well with an overall accuracy of 94 %. However, the measure of error is based on the normal distribution assumption, and data may not meet this assumption. Crossvalidation is a distribution free method, and may here be a more safe, and less biased approach to validation.

It performed very well, with errors mostly 0 and 1 out of 15 cases. We should add that Knime does not provide sensitivity and specificity measures here.

Note
More background, theoretical and mathematical information of validations and crossvalidations is given in:

Statistics Applied to Clinical Studies 5th Edition, Springer Heidelberg Germany.

Chap. 46 Validating qualitative diagnostic tests, pp. 509–517, 2012,

Chap. 47 Uncertainty of qualitative diagnostic tests, pp. 519–525, 2012,

Chap. 50 Validating quantitative diagnostic tests, pp. 545–552, 2012,

Chap. 51 Summary of validation procedures for diagnostic tests, pp. 555–568, 2012.

Machine Learning in Medicine Part One, Springer Heidelberg Germany.

Chap. 1 Introduction to machine learning, p. 5, 2012,

Chap. 3 Optimal scaling: discretization, p. 28, 2012,

Chap. 4 Optimal scaling, regularization including ridge, lasso, and elastic net regression, p. 41, 2012.

All of the above publications are from the same authors as the current work.

Chapter 17
Testing Parallel-Groups with Different Sample Sizes and Variances (5 Parallel-Group Studies)

17.1 General Purpose

Unpaired t-tests are traditionally used for testing the significance of difference between parallel-groups according to

$$t-value = (mean_1 - mean_2)/\sqrt{(SD_1/N_1 + SD_2/N_2)}$$

where mean, SD, N are respectively the mean, the standard deviation and the sample size of the parallel groups.

Many calculators on the internet (e.g., the P value calculator-GraphPad) can tell you whether the t-value is significantly smaller than 0.05, and, thus, whether there is a statistically significant difference between the parallel groups.

E.g., open Google and type p-value calculator for t-test...click Enter...click P value calculator-GraphPad...select P from t...t: enter computed t-value...DF: compute $N_1 + N_2 - 2$ and enter the result...click Compute P.

This procedure assumes that the two parallel groups have equal variances. However, in practice this is virtually never entirely true. This chapter is to assess tests accounting the effect of different variances on the estimated p-values.

17.2 Primary Scientific Question

Two methods for adjustment of different variances and different sample sizes are available, the pooled t-test which assumes that the differences in variances are just residual, and that the two variances are equal, and the Welch's test which assumes

© The Author(s) 2014
T.J. Cleophas and A.H. Zwinderman, *Machine Learning in Medicine—Cookbook Three*, SpringerBriefs in Statistics, DOI 10.1007/978-3-319-12163-5_17

that they are due to a real effect, like a difference in treatment effect with concomitant difference in spread of the data. How are the results of the two adjustment procedures.

17.3 Examples

In the underneath table the t-test statistics and *p*-values of 5 parallel-group studies with differences in the means, standard deviations (SDs) and sample sizes (Ns) are given. In the examples 2, 3, 4, and 5 respectively the Ns, SDs, means, and SDs have been changed as compared to example 1.

Means	SDs	Ns	Unadjusted		Adjusted (pooled)		Welch's adjust	
			t value	p value	t value	p value	t value	p value
1. 50/40	**5/3**	**100/200**	**1.715/0.087**		**1.811/0.071**		**1.715/0.088**	
2.		10/20	1.715/0.092		1.814/0.080		1.715/0.100	
3.	10/3		0.958/0.339		1.214/0.226		0.958/0.340	
4. 60/40			3.430/0.007		3.662/0.000		3.430/0.001	
5.	6/2		1.581/0.115		1.963/0.051		1.581/0.117	

Open Google and type GraphPad Software QuickCalcs t test calculator…mark: Enter mean, SEM, N…mark: Unpaired t test…label: type Group 1…mean: type 50…SEM: type 5…N: type 100…label: type Group 2… mean: type 40…SEM: type 3…N: type 200…click Calculate now.

In the output an adjusted t-value of 1.811 is given and a *p*-value of 0.071, slightly better than the unadjusted *p*-value of 0.087. Next a Welch's t-test will be performed using the same procedure as above, but with Welch's Unpaired t-test marked instead of just Unpaired t-test. The output sheet shows that the *p*-value is now worse than the unadjusted *p*-value instead of better.

In the examples 2–5 slightly different means, SDs, and Ns were used but, otherwise, the data were the same. After computations it can be observed that in all of the examples the adjusted test using pooled variances produced the best *p*-values. This sometimes lead to a statistically significant effect while the other two test are non-significant, for example with data 5 (*p*-value = 0.05). The Welch's adjustment produced the worst *p*-value, while the unadjusted produced the best statistics.

17.4 Conclusion

Two methods for adjustment of different variances and different sample sizes are available, the pooled t-test which assumes that the differences in variances are just residual, and the Welch's test which assumes that they are real differences. From 5 examples it can be observed that the t-tests using pooled variances consistently produced the best p-values sometimes leading to a statistically significant result in otherwise statistically insignificant data. In contrast, the Welch's adjustment consistently produced the worst result. The pooled t-test is probably the best option if we have clinical arguments for residual differences in variances, while the Welch's test would be a scientifically better option, if it can be argued that differences in variance were due to real clinical effects. Moreover, the Welch's test would be more in agreement with the general feature of advanced statistical analyses: tests taking special effects in the data into account are associated with larger p-values (more uncertainties).

Note

More background, theoretical and mathematical information of improved t-tests are in Statistics Applied to Clinical Studies, Chap. 2, The analysis of efficacy data, pp. 15–40, Springer Heidelberg Germany, 5th Edition, 2012, by the same authors.

Chapter 18
Association Rules Between Exposure and Outcome (50 and 60 Patients with Coronary Risk Factors)

18.1 General Purpose

Traditional analysis of exposure outcome relationships is only sensitive with strong relationships. This chapter is to assess whether association rules, based on conditional probabilities, may be more sensitive in case of weak relationships.

18.2 Primary Scientific Question

Is association rule analysis better sensitive than regression analysis and paired chi-square tests are for demonstrating significant exposure effects.

18.3 Example

The proportions observed in a sample are equal to chances or probabilities. If you observe a 40 % proportion of healthy patients, then the chance or probability (P) of being healthy in this group is 40 %. With two variables, e.g., healthy and happy, the symbol $\cap$ is often used to indicate "and" (both are present). Underneath a hypothesized example of 5 patients, with 3 of them having overweight and 2 of them coronary artery disease (CAD), is given.

© The Author(s) 2014
T.J. Cleophas and A.H. Zwinderman, *Machine Learning in Medicine—Cookbook Three*, SpringerBriefs in Statistics, DOI 10.1007/978-3-319-12163-5_18

Patient	Overweight (predictor)	Coronary artery disease
	X	Y
1	1	0
2	0	1
3	0	0
4	1	1
5	1	0

Support rule

$$\text{Support} = P\,X \cap Y = 1/5 = 0.2$$

Confidence rule

$$\text{Confidence} = P\,X \cap Y/P\,Y = [1/5]/[2/5] = 0.5$$

Lift rule (or lift-up rule)

$$\text{Lift} = P\,X \cap Y/[P\,X \times P\,Y] = [1/5]/[2/5 \times 2/5] = 1.25$$

Conviction rule

$$\text{Conviction} = [1 - P\,Y]/[1 - P\,X \cap Y/P\,Y] = [1 - 2/5]/[1 - 0.5] = 1.20$$

1. The support gives the proportion of patients with both overweight and CAD in the entire population. A support of 0.0 would mean that overweight and CAD are mutually elusive, a support of x · y would mean that the two factors are independent of one another.
2. The confidence gives the fraction of patients with both CAD and overweight in those with CAD. This fraction is obviously larger than that in the entire population, because it rose from 0.2 to 0.5.
3. The lift compares the observed proportion of patients with both overweight and CAD with the expected proportion if CAD and overweight would have occurred independently of one another. Obviously, the observed value is larger than expected, 1.25 versus 1.00, suggesting that overweight does contribute to the risk of CAD.
4. Finally, the conviction compares the patients with no-CAD in the entire population with those with both no-CAD and the presence of overweight. The ratio is larger than 1.00, namely 1.20. Obviously, the benefit of no-CAD is better for the entire population than it is for the subgroup with overweight.

In order to assess whether the computed values, like 0.2 and 1.25, are significantly different from 0.0 and 1.0 confidence intervals have to be calculated. We will use the McCallum-Layton calculator for proportions, freely available from the

Internet (Confidence interval calculator for proportions. www.mccallum-layton.co. uk/).

The calculations will somewhat overestimate the true confidence intervals, because the true confidence intervals are here mostly composed of two or more proportions, and this is not taken into account. Therefore, doubling the p-values may be more adequate (Bonferroni adjustment), but with very small p-values we need not worry.

18.3.1 Example One

A data set of 50 patients with coronary artery disease or not (1 = yes) and over-weight as predictor (1 = yes) is given underneath

Patient	Overweight	Coronary artery disease
1	1.00	0.00
2	0.00	1.00
3	0.00	0.00
4	1.00	1.00
5	0.00	0.00
6	1.00	0.00
7	0.00	1.00
8	0.00	0.00
9	1.00	1.00
10	0.00	0.00
11	1.00	0.00
12	0.00	1.00
13	0.00	0.00
14	1.00	1.00
15	0.00	0.00

The first 15 patients are given. The entire data file are the Variables A and B of the data file entitled "associationrule", and are in http://extras.springer.com.

20/50 of the patients have overweight (predictor), 20/50 have CAD. A paired binary test (McNemar's test) shows no significant difference between the two columns (p = 1.0). Binary logistic regression with the predictor as independent variable is equally insignificant (b = 0.69, p = 0.241).

Applying association rules we find a support of 0.2 and confidence of 0.5. The lift is 1.25 and the conviction is 1.20. The McCallum calculator gives the confi-dence intervals, respectively 10–34, 36–64, 110–145, and 107–137 %. All of these 95 % confidence intervals indicate a very significant difference from respectively

0 % (support and confidence) and 100 % (lift and conviction) with p-values < 0.001 (Bonferroni adjusted $p < 0.002$). Indeed, the predictor overweight had a very significant positive effect on the risk of CAD.

18.3.2 Example Two

A data set of 60 patients with coronary artery disease or not (1 = yes) with overweight and "being manager" as predictors (1 = yes)

Patient	Overweight	Manager	Coronary artery disease
1	1.00	1.00	0.00
2	0.00	0.00	1.00
3	1.00	1.00	0.00
4	0.00	1.00	1.00
5	0.00	0.00	0.00
6	1.00	1.00	1.00
7	1.00	1.00	0.00
8	0.00	0.00	1.00
9	1.00	1.00	0.00
10	0.00	1.00	1.00
11	0.00	0.00	0.00
12	1.00	1.00	1.00
13	1.00	1.00	0.00
14	0.00	0.00	1.00
15	1.00	1.00	0.00

The first 15 patients are given. The entire data file are the variables C, D, and E of the data file entitled "associationrule", and is in http://extras.springer.com.

Instead of a single x-variable now 2 of them are included. 30/60 of the patients have overweight, 40/60 are manager, and 30/60 have CAD. A paired binary test (Cochran's test) shows no significant difference between the three columns ($p = 0.082$). Binary logistic regression with the two predictors as independent variables is equally insignificant (b-values are—21.9 and 21.2, p-values are 0.99 and 0.99).

Applying association rules we find a support of 0.1666 and confidence of 0.333. The lift is 2.0 and the conviction is 1.25. The McCallum calculator gives the confidence intervals. Expressed as percentages they are respectively, 8–29, 22–47, and 159–270 and 108–136 %. All of these 95 % confidence intervals indicate a very significant difference from respectively 0 % (support and confidence) and 100 % (lift and conviction) with p-values <0.001 (Bonferroni adjusted $p < 0.002$ or <0.003). Indeed, the predictors overweight and being manager had a statistically very significant effect on the risk of CAD.

18.4 Conclusion

Association rule analysis is more sensitive than regression analysis and paired chi-square tests, and is able to demonstrate significant predictor effects, when the other methods are not. It can also include multiple variables and very large datasets and is a welcome methodology for clinical predictor research.

Note

More background, theoretical and mathematical information of association rules are in Machine Learning in Medicine Part Two, Chap. 11, pp. 105–113, Springer Heidelberg Germany, 2013, by the same authors.

Chapter 19
Confidence Intervals for Proportions and Differences in Proportions

19.1 General Purpose

Proportions, fractions, percentages, risks, hazards are all synonymous terms to indicate what part of a population had events like death, illness, complications etc. Instead of p-values, confidence intervals are often calculated. If you obtained many samples from the same population, 95 % of them would have their mean results between the 95 % confidence intervals. And, likewise, samples from the same population with their proportions outside the 95 % confidence intervals means that they are significantly different from the population with a probability of 5 % ($p < 0.05$). This chapter is to assess how confidence intervals can be computed.

19.2 Primary Scientific Question

P-values give the type I error, otherwise called the chance of finding a difference where there is none. Confidence intervals tell you the same, but, in addition, they give the range in which the true outcome value lies, and the direction and strength of it. Are confidence intervals more relevant for exploratory studies than p-values, because of the additional information provided.

© The Author(s) 2014
T.J. Cleophas and A.H. Zwinderman, *Machine Learning in Medicine—Cookbook Three*, SpringerBriefs in Statistics, DOI 10.1007/978-3-319-12163-5_19

19.3 Example

If in two parallel groups of respectively 100 and 75 patients the numbers of patients with an event are 75 and 50, according to a z-test or chi-square test (see Statistics Applied to Clinical Studies Fifth Edition, Chap. 3, The analysis of safety data, pp. 41–60, 2012, Springer Heidelberg Germany, from the same authors), then the *p*-value of difference will be 0.23. This means that we have 23 % chance of a type one error, and that this chance is far too large to be statistically significant ($p > 0.05$).

In the two above groups the proportions are respectively $75/100 = 0.750$ and $50/75 = 0.667$. The standard errors of these proportions can be calculated from the equation

$$\text{standard errors} = \pm\sqrt{(p(1-p)/\sqrt{n})}$$

where p = proportion and n = sample size.

$$95\,\%\ \text{confidence intervals} = \pm1.96\sqrt{(p(1-p)/\sqrt{n})}$$

If you have little affinity with computations, then plenty of calculators on the internet are helpful.

19.3.1 Confidence Intervals of Proportions

We will use the free "Matrix Software". Open Google and type Standard Error (SE) of Sample Proportion Calculator-Binomial Standard Deviation...click Enter...click Matrix Software...in Calculate SE Sample Proportion of Standard deviation type 0.75 for Proportion of successes (p)...type 100 for Number of Observations (n)... click Calculate...

The binomial SE of the Sample proportion $= \pm0.04330127$
The 95 % confidence interval of this proportion $= \pm1.96 \times 0.04330127$
$$= \pm0.08487$$
$$= \text{between } 0.66513 \text{ and } 0.83487$$

Similarly the 95 % confidence interval of the data from group 2 can be calculated.

19.3.2 Confidence Intervals of Differences in Proportions

In order to calculate the confidence interval of the differences between the above two proportions, we will use the free Vassarstats. Open Google and type http://vassarstats.net/prop2_ind.html...click enter...select The Confidence Interval for the Difference Between Two Independent Proportions...Larger Proportion: k_a (number of observations with event) =: type 75...n_a (total number of observations) =: type 100...click Calculate.

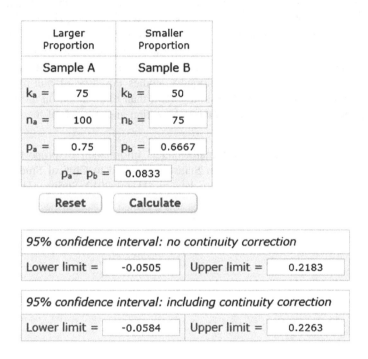

The output is given above. p_a and p_b are the proportions, $p_a - p_b$ the difference. The 95 % confidence interval is between −0.0505 and 0.2183.

Proportions are yes/no data, e.g., a proportion of 75 subjects out of 100 had an event. The normal distribution is used for the calculation of the p-values and confidence intervals. In order to test yes/no data with a normal distribution, a continuity correction can be used to improve the quality of the analysis. In the example given the 75/100 in your sample indicates that the real event rate in your entire population of, e.g., 1,000 may be between 745 and 755/1,000. Because 745/1,000 is, of course, smaller than 750/1,000, it would make sense to use the proportion 745/1,000 for the calculation of the confidence interval instead of 750/1,000. This procedure is called the continuity correction, and as shown above it produces somewhat wider confidence intervals, and, thus, more uncertainty in your data. Unfortunately, higher quality is often associated with larger levels of uncertainty.

19.4 Conclusion

Proportions are used to indicate what part of a population had events. Instead of p-values to tell you whether your observed proportion is statistically significantly different from a proportion of 0.0, 95 % confidence intervals are often calculated. If you obtained many samples from the same population, 95 % of them would have their result between the 95 % confidence intervals. And, likewise, samples from the same population having their proportions outside the 95 % confidence intervals means that they are significantly different from the population with a probability of 5 % ($p < 0.05$). P-values give the type I error, otherwise called the chance of finding a difference where there is none, or the chance of erroneously rejecting the null-hypothesis. Confidence intervals tell you the same, but, in addition, they give you the range in which the true outcome value lies, and the direction and strength of it. Particularly, for data mining of exploratory studies the issue of null-hypothesis testing with p-values is generally less important than information on the range in which the true outcome value lies, and the direction and strength of it.

Note

More background, theoretical and mathematical information of proportions and their confidence intervals is given in Statistics Applied to Clinical Studies Fifth Edition, Chap. 3, The analysis of safety data, pp. 41–60, 2012, Springer Heidelberg Germany, from the same authors.

Chapter 20
Ratio Statistics for Efficacy Analysis of New Drugs (50 Patients Treated for Hypercholesterolemia)

20.1 General Purpose

Treatment efficacies are often assessed as differences from baseline. However, better treatment efficacies may be observed in patients with high baseline-values than in those with low ones. This was, e.g., the case in the Progress study, a parallel-group study of pravastatin versus placebo (see Statistics Applied to Clinical Studies Fifth Edition, Chap. 17, Logistic and Cox regression, Markov models, and Laplace transformations, pp. 199–218, Springer Heidelberg Germany, 2012, from the same authors). This chapter assesses the performance of ratio statistics for that purpose.

20.2 Primary Scientific Question

The differences of treatment efficacy and baseline may be the best fit test statistic, if the treatment efficacies are independent of baseline. However, if not, then ratios of the two may fit the data better.

© The Author(s) 2014
T.J. Cleophas and A.H. Zwinderman, *Machine Learning in Medicine—Cookbook Three*, SpringerBriefs in Statistics, DOI 10.1007/978-3-319-12163-5_20

20.3 Example

A 50-patient 5-group parallel-group study was performed with 5 different choles-
terol-lowering compounds. The first 12 patients of the data file is underneath. The
entire data file is entitled "ratiostatistics" and is in http://extras.springer.com.

Variable			
1	2	3	4
Baseline	Treatment	Treatment	Baseline minus treatment
Cholesterol (mmol/l)	Cholesterol (mmol/l)	Group no.	Cholesterol level (mmol/l)
6.10	5.20	1.00	0.90
7.00	7.90	1.00	−0.90
8.20	3.90	1.00	4.30
7.60	4.70	1.00	2.90
6.50	5.30	1.00	1.20
8.40	5.40	1.00	3.00
6.90	4.20	1.00	2.70
6.70	6.10	1.00	0.60
7.40	3.80	1.00	3.60
5.80	6.30	1.00	−0.50
6.20	4.30	2.00	1.90
7.10	6.80	2.00	0.30

Start by opening the above data file in SPSS statistical software.

Command:
Graphs…Legacy Dialogs…Error Bar…mark Summaries of groups of cases…
click Define…Variable: enter "baseline minus treatment"…Category Axis: enter
Treatment group…Confidence interval for mean: Level enter 95 %…click OK.

The underneath graph shows that all of the treatments were excellent and significantly lowered cholesterol levels as shown by the 95 % confidence intervals. T-
tests are not needed here.

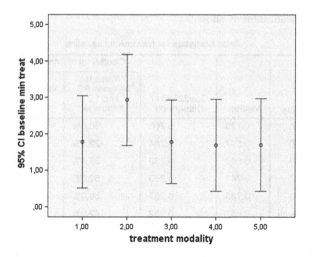

A one-way ANOVA (treatment modality as predictor and "baseline minus treatment" as outcome) will be performed to assess whether any of the treatments significantly outperformed the others.

Command:
Analyze...Compare means...One-Way ANOVA...Dependent List: enter "baseline minus treatment"...Factor: enter Treatment group...click OK.

ANOVA

baseline min treat

	Sum of Squares	df	Mean Square	F	Sig.
Between Groups	10.603	4	2.651	0.886	0.480
Within Groups	134.681	45	2.993		
Total	145.284	49			

According to the above table the differences between the different treatment were statistically insignificant. And, so, according to the above analysis all treatments were excellent and no significance difference between any of the groups were observed. Next, we will try and find out whether ratio statistics can make additional observations.

Command:
Analyze...Descriptive Statistics...Ratio...Numerator: enter "treatment"... Denominator: enter "baseline"...Group Variable: enter "treatmentmodality (treatment group)"...click Statistics...mark Median...mark COD (coefficient of dispersion)...Concentration Index: Low Proportion: type 0.8...High Proportion: type 1.2...click Add...Percent of Median: enter 20...click Add...click Continue...click OK.

The underneath table is shown.

Ratio Statistics for treatment / baseline

			Coefficient of Concentration	
Group	Median	Coefficient of Dispersion	Percent between 0.8 and 1.2 inclusive	Within 20% of Median inclusive
1.00	0.729	0.265	50.0%	50.0%
2.00	0.597	0.264	22.2%	44.4%
3.00	0.663	0.269	36.4%	54.5%
4.00	0.741	0.263	50.0%	50.0%
5.00	0.733	0.267	50.0%	50.0%
Overall	0.657	0.282	42.0%	38.0%

A problem with ratios is, that they usually suffer from overdispersion, and, therefore, the spread in the data must be assessed differently from that of normal distributions. First medians are applied, which is not the mean value but the values in the middle of all values. Assessment of spread is then estimated with

(1) the coefficient of dispersion,
(2) the percentual coefficient of concentration (all ratios within 20 % of the median are included),
(3) the interval coefficient of concentration (all ratios between the ratio 0.8 * median and 1.2 * median are included (* = symbol of multiplication).

The coefficients (2) and (3) are not the same, if the distribution of the ratios are very skewed.

The above table shows the following.

Treatment 1 (Group 1) performs best with 60 % reduction of cholesterol after treatment, treatment 4 performs worst with only 74 % reduction of cholesterol after treatment. The coefficient (1) is a general measure of variability of the ratios and the coefficient (3) shows the same but is more easy to interpret: around 50 % of the individual ratios are within 20 % distance from the median ratio. The coefficient (2) gives the percentage of individual ratios between the interval of 0.8 and 1.2 * median ratio. Particularly, groups 2 and 3 have small coefficients indicating little concentration of the individual ratios here. Group 2 may produce the best median ratio, but is also least concentrated, and is thus more uncertain than, e.g., groups 1, 4, 5.

It would make sense to conclude from these observations that treatment group 1 with more certainty is a better treatment choice than treatment group 2.

20.4 Conclusion

Treatment efficacies are often assessed as differences from baseline. However, better treatment efficacies may be observed in patients with high baseline-values than in those with low ones. The differences of treatment efficacy and baseline may be the best fit test statistic, if the treatment efficacies are independent of baseline. However, if not, then ratios of the two may fit the data better, and allow for relevant additional conclusions.

Note
More background, theoretical and mathematical information of treatment efficacies that are not independent of baseline is given in Statistics Applied to Clinical Studies Fifth Edition, Chap. 17, Logistic and Cox regression, Markov models, and Laplace transformations, pp. 199–218, Springer Heidelberg Germany, 2012, from the same authors.

Index

© The Author(s) 2014
T.J. Cleophas and A.H. Zwinderman, *Machine Learning in Medicine—Cookbook Three*, SpringerBriefs in Statistics, DOI 10.1007/978-3-319-12163-5